The Stories Behind the Poses

First published in 2022 by Leaping Hare Press,
an imprint of The Quarto Group.
The Old Brewery, 6 Blundell Street
London, N7 9BH,
United Kingdom
T (0)20 7700 6700
www.Quarto.com

A catalogue record for this book is available from the British Library.

ISBN 978-0-7112-7188-3
Ebook ISBN 978-0-7112-7189-0

10 9 8 7 6 5 4 3 2 1

Commissioning editor Chloe Murphy
Design by Ginny Zeal and Isabel Eeles
With special thanks to Dr. Layne Little

MIX
Paper from responsible sources
FSC® C016973

Printed in China

The yoga poses depicted in this book are included solely the purposes of referencing the stories behind them and are not intended as recommendations or instructions for the performance of physical yoga. Before performing any physical yoga, the reader should fully inform themselves and consult with a qualified yoga instructor and with the reader's medical practitioner. Information given in this book is not intended to be taken as a replacement for physical or mental health advice and any person with a condition requiring medical attention should consult a qualified medical practitioner or therapist. The publisher and the author make no representations or warranties with respect to the accuracy or completeness of the contents of this book, and specifically disclaim, without limitation, any implied warranties of fitness for a particular purpose and exclude all liability to the extent permitted by law for any injury, illness, damage, liability, or loss incurred, directly or indirectly, from the use or application of any of the contents of this book.

The Stories Behind the Poses

THE INDIAN MYTHOLOGY
THAT INSPIRED
50 YOGA
POSTURES

DR. RAJ BALKARAN

ILLUSTRATED BY DEVIKA MENON

Leaping Hare Press

INTRODUCTION

THE POWER OF STORY

Storytelling is no ordinary thing. It is how we make sense of the world. While science is surely the arbiter of the empirical world, storytelling is most certainly the medium of making sense of that world. From mythic stories, to life stories, to news stories, storytelling is a perennially human affair. Stories communicate, elucidate, and persuade at every turn, and there is perhaps no more powerful a teaching tool than storytelling.

Myth is pitched between heaven and earth. It is the most potent, profound, and pervasive form of storytelling. Some consider mythology as history, while others consider it as fantasy. Irrespective, myths are tools for making meaning, most importantly about what it means to be human. Myths mirror the complexities of life. They are maps for the human journey and, as dramatizations of the inner life, they broach life's big questions and life's mysteries. They accomplish important work in the quiet periphery of our conscious awareness, humming away in the background, as they celebrate the human spirit, and form the bedrock of culture and the human psyche.

THE STORIES BEHIND THE POSES

Perhaps nowhere more so is the power of mythology more evident than in the Indic context. Indian thought, art, song, dance, and ritual are inextricable from Indian myth. While few know the content of ancient Indian ritual and philosophy, everyone across the Indic world knows the stories from the Sanskrit Epics and Purāṇas, from which this book draws.

These are India's "tales of old", featuring gods and kings, and wondrous things. They are captivating, insightful, and immensely didactic in nature. The universe of Indian myth is populated with faces of divinity, sages, gods, nymphs, and kings. It is a space of sacred places, multiple realms, and cyclical time where the universe is created, sustained, dissolved, and recreated ad infinitum. It is a space where divine power can be harnessed through devotion and arduous penance, and used for good and ill alike.

These stories offer a window into the system of values and beliefs that pervade the Indic world, and it is from these stories that yoga hails. Yoga is an ancient banyan tree, one nourished by Indic soil—and the bedrock of Indian tradition is found in Indian myth.

WHO IS THIS BOOK FOR?

This book is for seekers and lovers of stories. It is also for those who wish to deepen their yoga practice. It is a resource for students, lifelong learners, and avid yoga practitioners, as it delves into the rich mythology underpinning 50 yoga poses to elucidate the philosophical truths to be found within them.

My hope is that this book will not only deepen your inner life, but will also introduce you to and inspire you to learn more about the lore of ancient India, from where yoga stems, and the profound life wisdom it encodes.

While this book will certainly enhance your spiritual yoga practice, please note that it should not be used to establish a physical practice. The practice of postural yoga is best done in the care of a trusted yoga teacher, in tandem with expert medical consultancy on a yoga practice that supports your specific physical, emotional, and mental needs.

HOW TO USE THIS BOOK

This book tells the stories behind 50 yoga poses as found in Indian myth. For each pose, I have shared with you my own telling of each story, and included a passage at the end of each to break down the lessons of the pose, and help you embody these teachings in your life and in your yoga practice.

I have also highlighted three key themes of each tale to help you better understand their teachings, as well as to help you plan a themed yoga class into which you can incorporate the pose, its teachings, and its story.

If you are a yoga teacher, consider enhancing your class's experience by reading a story of your choice aloud to your class, and call to mind the themes of the story while teaching its pertinent posture. If you are a solo yoga practitioner, consider reading one story before or after class to set the stage for your practice, or close your practice, as you tap into the themes of the story for your personal growth as a yogī.

Above and beyond facilitating a physical posture, the stories told in this book are aimed at aligning one's inner positioning, orienting one toward personal growth and yogic aspirations. Rather than being seated on a mat, these myths are seated in the play of consciousness. These stories are meant to be lived and relived within your heart so that you may embody the wisdom they encode.

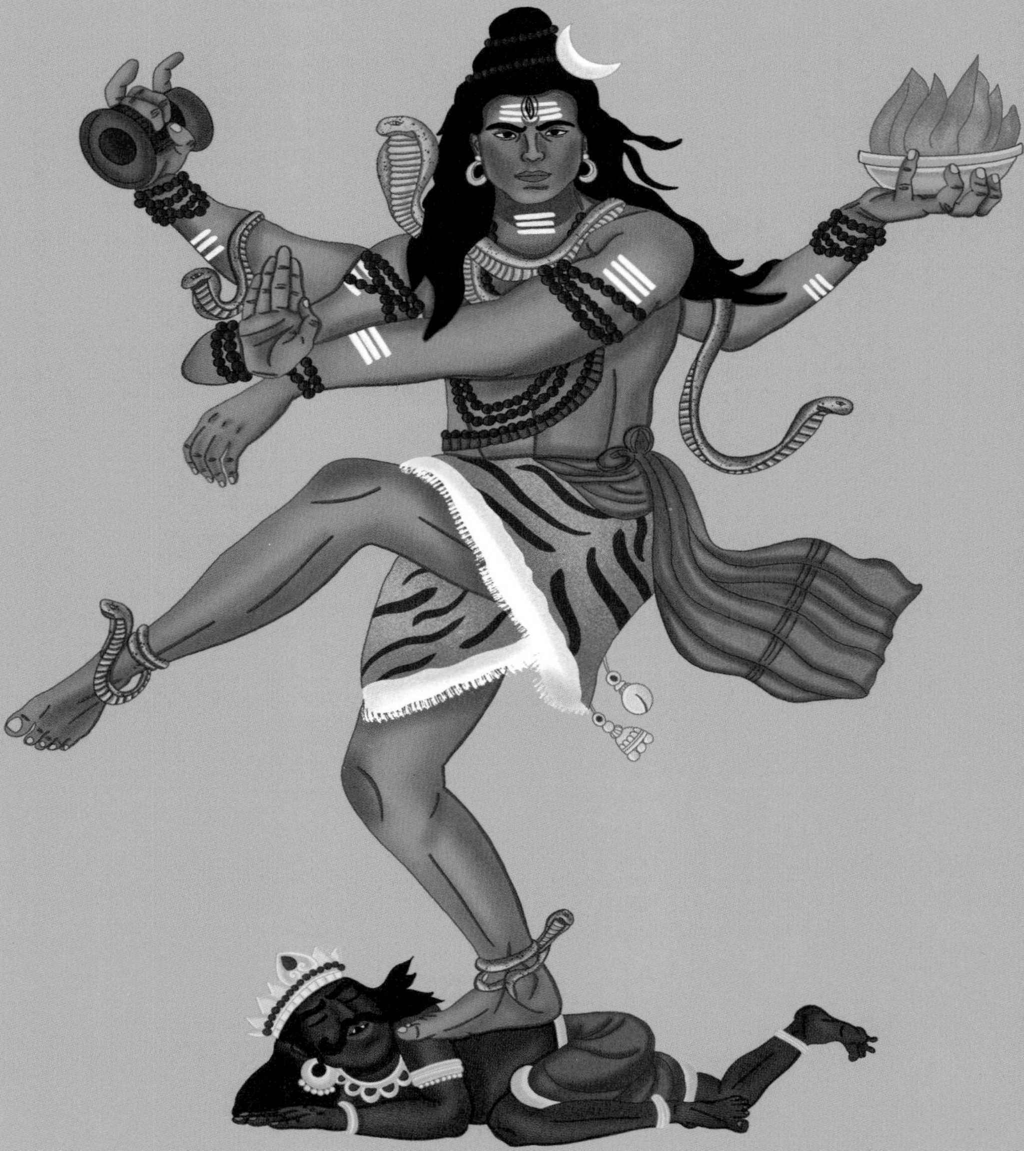

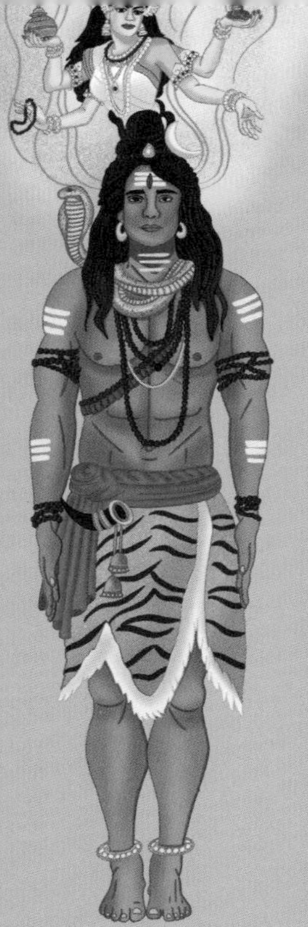

CHAPTER 1

Śiva, Lord of Yoga

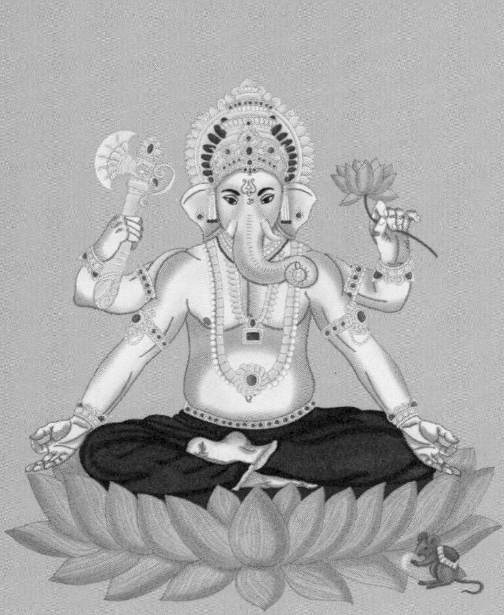

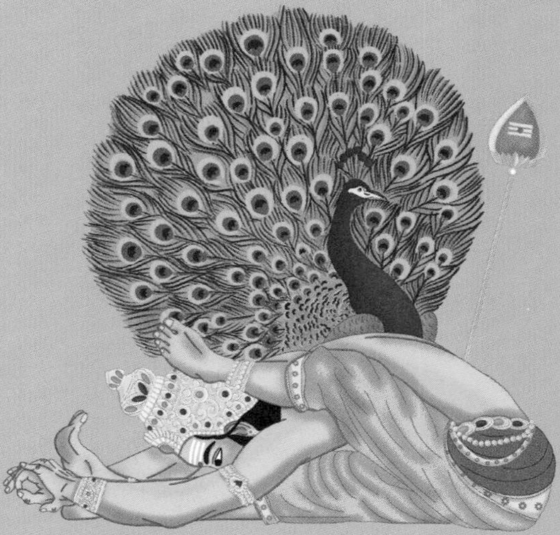

PERFECTION POSE

SIDDHĀSANA

THE POWER OF YOGIC MEDITATION

THEMES
Wisdom
Insight
Awareness

LONG AGO, WHEN THE AGE WAS YOUNG, the Brahmin priests were performing rituals for the welfare of the world. They were wise, and understood the importance of auspicious beginnings—that how a thing begins can often color the way that it turns out. They rightly emphasized the importance of starting a relationship on the right foot, or getting up on the right side of the bed. So, a very important question arose: Who among the gods should be worshipped first? They completed a fire sacrifice to the great lord Śiva whereby, along with special herbs and clarified butter, their intention to learn which god should be worshipped before all others was carried up to Śiva's abode. The prayer entered the mind of Śiva, and so he interrupted his meditation to visit and consult with his consort, Pārvatī, the wise earth goddess. Pārvatī was delighted to see him, and even more so to learn of his inquiry.

"Well," she said with a glint in her eye and an air of mystery in her smile, "surely it should be one of our two sons, Kārttikeya or Gaṇeśa. They contain the best of us!"

Śiva agreed that this was an excellent idea, and the two of them agreed that whichever of their sons could prove himself worthy would be the rightful recipient of the honor.

"But how will we determine which of them is more worthy?" Śiva wondered aloud.

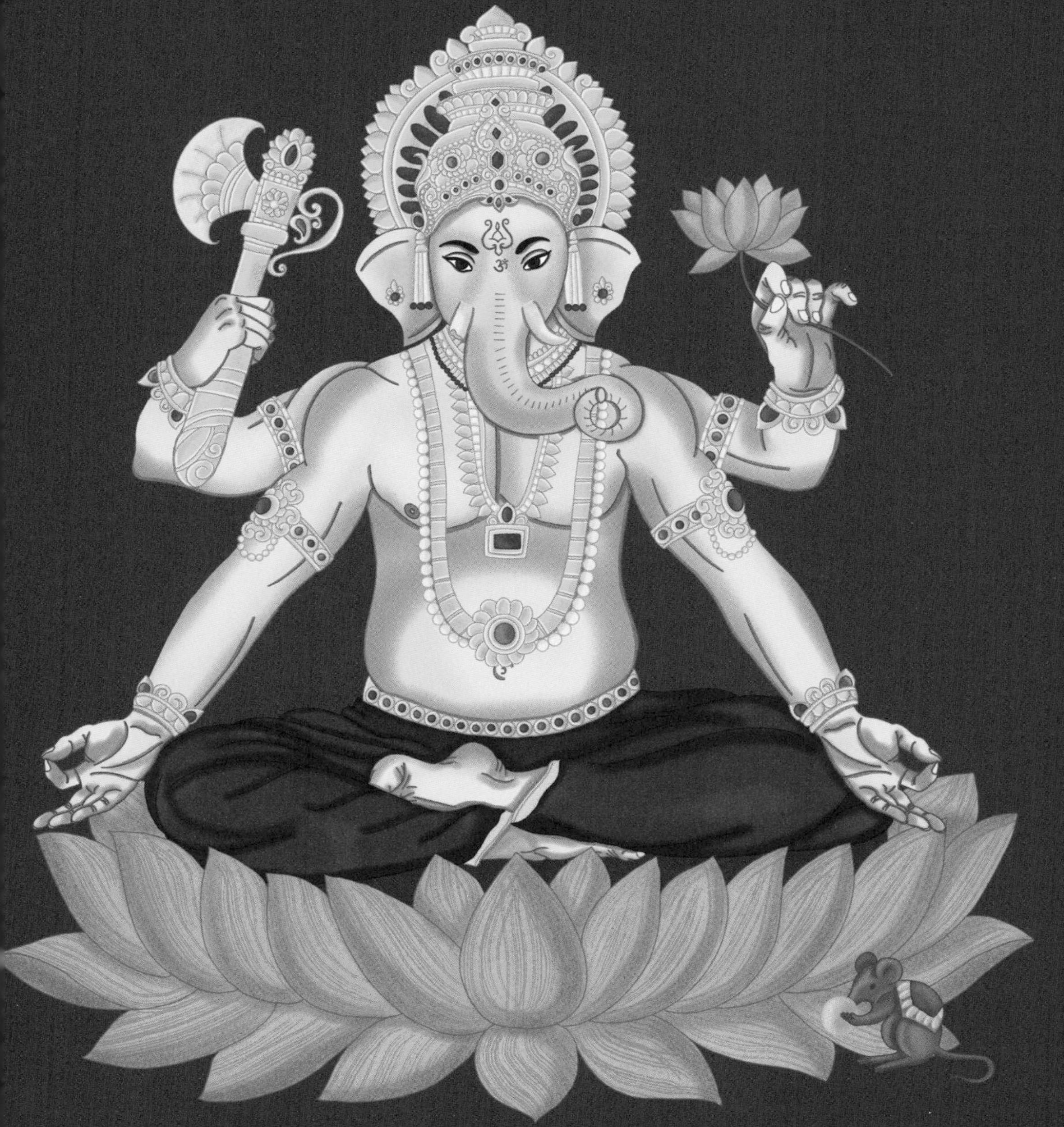

Pārvatī already had the answer on the tip of her tongue. "How about a race?" she suggested with a widening smile.

Śiva instantly took a liking to the idea. Becoming visibly excited, he asked, "But a race from where to where?"

"It seems to me," she asserted, "that for such an important prize, it would be only fitting for them to race around Earth itself." As she proposed the idea, Śiva remembered why he adored her as he did:

"You are as wise as you are beautiful, my love."

The sons of Śiva and Pārvatī were summoned and given their instructions. They were to race around the world to decide which of them would henceforth be considered foremost among all gods. The second Śiva signalled the start of the race, Kārttikeya, the proud Commander of the Celestial Army was off, riding his peacock, swift as lightning, over the horizon in the blink of an eye. Pārvatī and Śiva were in awe at his speed, and so too was Gaṇeśa. The round-bellied Lord of Wisdom was certain that the goddess had favored his brother, for how could he be expected to compete, riding a mouse? Though he was not feeling competitive, he knew he had to fullfill his duty somehow. So, he collected himself, took a deep breath and turned inward. After a moment of reflection, inspiration struck. He looked over at his parents Śiva and Pārvatī, resplendent, shining like the sun and moon sharing the sky, and reverently circled them. Once, twice, three times. He then returned to his meditative posture, connected with the grounding energy of the mountains, enjoying the blissful peace within his being.

Before long, Kārttikeya returned, triumphant, exhilarated, eager to claim his prize, seeing that Gaṇeśa had not yet even departed! Śiva and Pārvatī were proud of his feat and Śiva was about to declare his victory, but Pārvatī, with her characteristic air of delicate and enticing mystery, suggested they first check in with Gaṇeśa before proceeding.

"Gaṇeśa, you're always so obedient, so steadfast, so dependable! Why did you not do your duty and race with your brother?" Śiva questioned.

"Father, it is clear to me that our divine mother has favored my brother on this day, for how could I possibly compete with him in this race around the world? But I knew I had to fullfill my duty somehow. Having turned inward for inspiration, I decided to encircle you both. Upon my first circumambulation, I was taken with the powerful presence of the goddess, our mother, whose divine play creates the world about us. She is the energy of name and form on which our very experiences are based! Then I was inspired to encircle again, and I saw that you, father, are the divine consciousness behind all things. Upon my third and final circumambulation, I saw into the mystery of your divine union, where consciousness and energy are two sides of the cosmic coin, where there was no difference between the two of you, nor between you two and me, nor among the world and all beings within it! I am content to concede victory to my brother, Kārttikeya, the swift!"

Śiva and Pārvatī were more than satisfied that Gaṇeśa had done his duty, and Śiva addressed his elder son, "Arise, Kārttikeya, and claim your title!"

"Father, I cannot. For, the goddess did favor one of us upon this day, but my victory here is mere illusion. It is Gaṇeśa who has won this race, for, while I encircled the decaying, impermanent globe, he encircled imperishable truth, which is within us all. I would give a thousand victories for an ounce of the wisdom that my brother possesses."

Śiva glowed with pride as he looked over at the goddess. Even now, he could not be sure how much of the day's events she had planned all along. But he would have eons to contemplate her divine mysteries once the task at hand had been completed. So he called to his second son: "Arise, Gaṇeśa, Remover of Obstacles, Wisdom Incarnate. I declare that from this day until I bring destruction upon this world, you shall be first among the gods! In every temple, in every home, at every festival, ritual, and practice, let no sacrifice be accepted, let no blessing be conferred lest you be invoked first, from now until the end of time. For how can anyone succeed lest they commence with wisdom? Arise, Gaṇeśa, son of Śiva and Pārvatī, foremost of the gods!"

The wisdom of Gaṇeśa resides in taking the time to calmly look inside before rushing headlong into action. Though it may seem difficult to find time for meditation and yoga practice amidst the busyness of our lives, this story shows us why it must nonetheless be pursued. The physical practice of yoga is ultimately an exercise in the embodiment of the divine interplay of Śiva and Pārvatī; a way for us to inhabit the body that affords us the insight into the relationship between these cosmic principles. When you sit in Siddhāsana, contemplate the wisdom of Gaṇeśa and remember the divine play that lies at the heart of your own being.

ELEPHANT TRUNK POSE

EKA-HASTA-BHUJĀSANA

GAṆEŚA, SON OF ŚIVA

THEMES
Surrender
Balance
Grounding

THE MARRIAGE OF PĀRVATĪ AND ŚIVA, though blessed, was never simple. As much as Śiva adored Pārvatī, his first love was yoga. He was always off meditating, seeking higher and higher levels of attainment. And though she loved him with all her heart, waiting for eons on end for Śiva to complete his meditative practices was difficult for Pārvatī. She knew better than to disrupt his trances, but on one occasion, after a millennium or two had elapsed, her loneliness got the better of her and she longed for a child. She scratched a bit of skin from her arm, and with it crafted a son whom she named Gaṇeśa. Such is the power of the divine feminine, the source of all life, the creatrix of all things. Hers is the power of *māyā*, of magic, of manifestation. She mystically produced her son from her own body. The feminine is the primordial—it comes first.

Pārvatī was deeply at home in motherhood, and she was overjoyed. Not only was she the mother of all creation, but now she had a child to call her own, a point of focus for the full breadth of her oceanic love. In the blink of an eye, Gaṇeśa grew through boyhood and into his youth. He was devoted to his mother, so when she called on him one day to guard their home, while she bathed in the river by the mountainside behind their abode, he was proud. "Make sure no one trespasses while I am gone," she said to her son, and

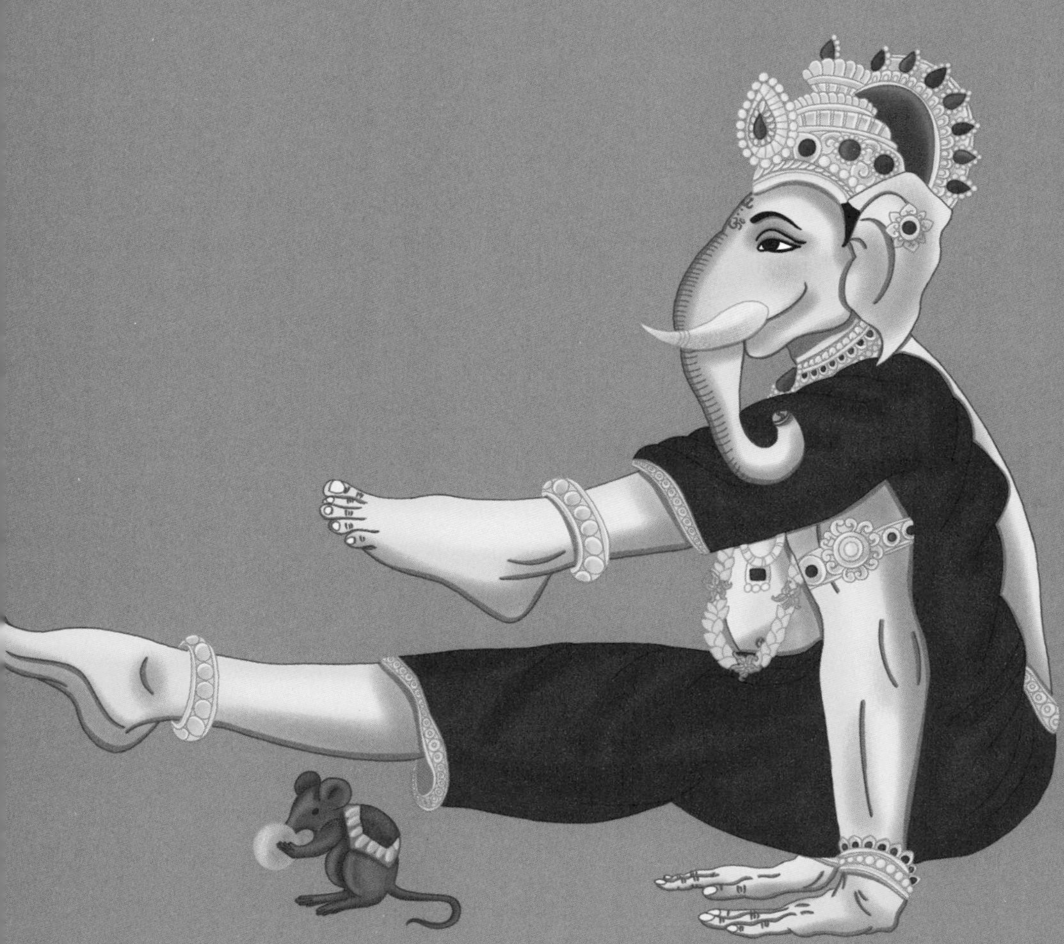

he gladly assented, "None shall pass!" The goddess smiled lovingly and disappeared out of sight.

As fate would have it, at that very moment, the mountains rumbled as Śiva, the great Yogī, awoke from his divine trance. As his awareness returned to his body, he arose, and his mind turned to thinking of his beautiful wife. He eagerly descended unto his abode, expecting to find her there. But as he approached, he noticed a rather haughty looking youth standing to attention at the entrance. Śiva commanded him to step aside but Gaṇeśa replied, "You cannot pass!" Śiva tried for a second time: "Step aside!" he shouted, but Gaṇeśa was steadfast, intent on guarding his mother's abode, replying, "You cannot pass!" In the blink of an eye, Śiva pulled out his sword, decapitated the arrogant lad, breathed a sigh of relief to be done with that nonsense, and entered his abode.

Pārvatī had finished her bath out back just as Śiva arrived, and was delighted to see him. They embraced in divine ecstasy, and Pārvatī excitedly proclaimed, "Śiva, my darling, I am so glad you're home! And you've had a chance to meet our son! He was guarding the front door for me when you arrived!"

Śiva knew that he had no choice but to tell his wife what had happened. Pārvatī was devastated and enraged, and demanded that he go out immediately into the world and find a replacement head for their son. So, Śiva departed, in pensive mood, reflecting upon his tendencies toward violent outbursts.

As he wondered the countryside, ruminating on past mistakes, Śiva came across an elephant. His first instinct was to simply lop the creature's head off, but as he approached it, he caught himself in the sudden glare of his own awareness. He reined himself in, knowing that this time, he must take a more measured approach, a nd break the habit of decapitating first and facing the consequences later. So, Śiva explained his plight to the attentive elephant, who responded with astonishing composure:

"Is that all, Lord Śiva? By all means then, please sever my head and install it on your son's body."

"You would so willingly surrender your life, Elephant?" Śiva asked.

"I have lived a long time, Lord, and learned a lot in all that time. Death is certain for all creatures in the goddess' creation. You offer me the opportunity to live on as part of your son. This is a rare chance indeed, and far more than any elephant could dream of. Please accept my head in grateful service."

Śiva was so humbled that he blessed the elephant, liberating him from rebirth, as he accepted his offering, and returned to his abode. He affixed the head of the elephant to the body of his son and breathed new life into him. Gaṇeśa opened his eyes, his vision was clear and calm, supported by the wisdom of the great elephant. He now saw what he could not see before; he recognized Śiva for the great lord that he was, and asked for forgiveness for his arrogance. Śiva in turn asked forgiveness for his own mistake. The goddess beamed, and all rejoiced in her mystery and majesty, in the divine play whereby both her husband and son learned humility, graced by the wisdom of the elephant.

When we surrender our mundane heads to be divinely decapitated, as the elephant does in this story, we see through the goddess' material play and can recognize the spirit of Śiva wherever we go. Śiva and the goddess are ultimately one, two sides of the same cosmic coin, but separate in order to experience the ecstasy of uniting. Deluded by materiality, we see others as separate from ourselves, like a head separated from a body. But when blessed with the vision of the wise, we see separation as the illusion that blocks the light of spiritual union.

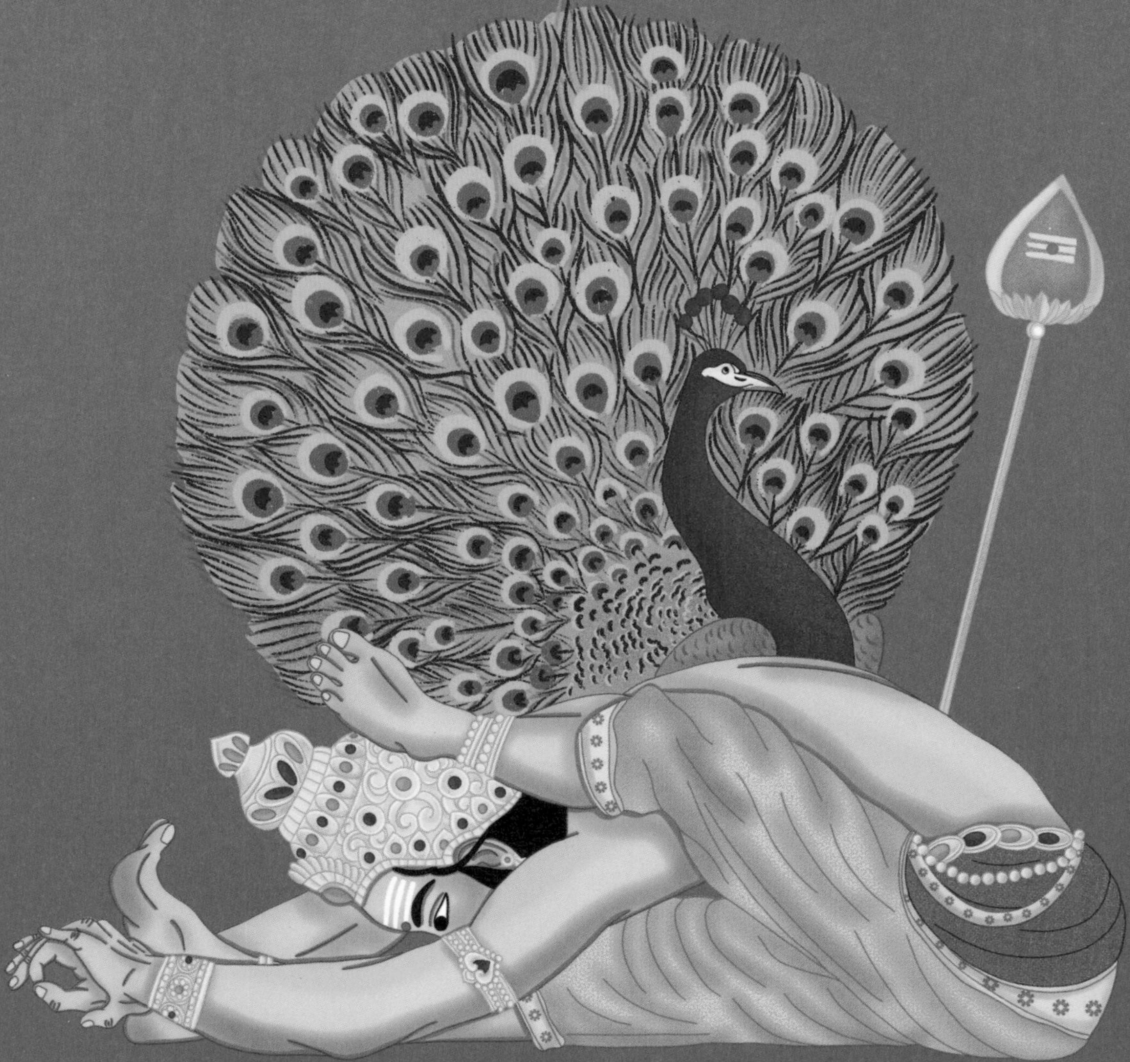

WAR GOD POSE
SKANDĀSANA

SKANDA,
SON OF ŚIVA

THEMES
Grounding
Respect
Attention

Long ago, a great demon named Taraka once terrorized the heavens. King Indra and his entourage of gods were greatly disturbed at the prospect of losing their sovereignty and having their heavenly abode usurped by Taraka and his hordes. In their despair, they went to Lord Brahmā, Grandfather of Creation, for guidance.

"You must do something, Grandfather Brahmā! Taraka is a creature of your creation, so surely you must know how to stop him!"

"Indeed, I do," replied Lord Brahmā, "since it was none other than me who granted him invincibility."

"What!" exclaimed the gods, "It was you who made him so powerful? But why?"

"Well, it was, and it wasn't me. Let me explain. Do you think this universe of mine sustains itself through arbitrary randomness? No. It is governed by certain principles, the most crucial of which is karma—as you sow, so shall you reap. Taraka had performed thousands of years of penance, and so he was owed a boon. He earned it by virtue of this sacred law. Demons such as he always ask for immortality. You gods may hoard the Elixir of Immortality for yourselves. Nonetheless, the demons always desire to be your equal, and enjoy everlasting life, as you do. Of course, I cannot give them absolute immortality, but when I asked Taraka what boon he wanted, he declared, 'make me invincible to all except for the child produced by Śiva's seed!' I had no choice but to grant his boon, which was very clever, as the great Yogī never spills his seed!"

The gods gasped. Their predicament seemed all the worse. "What do we do then, Grandfather?"

"Is no one listening to me? Only a child spawned by Śiva's seed can destroy Taraka."

"But how do we possibly get Śiva to spawn a child?"

"You'll have to devise a plan to do so! You're much more than mere puppets in this creation of mine. I've explained the principles at play, so go ahead and sort it out as you will! Now please excuse me while I return to my meditation."

The gods devised a plan. Although Śiva was a celibate ascetic, the gods were well aware that Pārvatī, the daughter of the mountains, was truly in love with him, and wanted nothing more than to be his wife. So, one day, when Pārvatī was walking in the hills, close to Śiva's abode, beautifully clad, scented, and shining like the rising moon, the gods dispatched Kāma, the god of erotic desire. Kāma aimed his amorous arrows at Śiva just at the moment that Pārvatī was walking by. Śiva's eyes fluttered open and he desired nothing more than to be with Pārvatī. He soon realized Kāma's role in all of this, and ended up reducing Kāma to ashes. Śiva oscillated between eons in cosmic trance, and eons of divine rapture in Pārvatī's loving embrace. But still, Śiva saved his seed to garner spiritual power, rather than spill it for physical pleasure. So, the gods had to devise yet another plan.

They dispatched the fire god, Agni, in the guise of a peacock to intervene in the celestial couple's amorous affairs. Agni perched on the branch of a tree just outside of Śiva and Pārvatī's home, awaiting the commencement of their divine union. At the height of their passion, he let out a sharp call while fanning his tail to majestic fullness. The distraction was so great that Śiva lost focus and climaxed. Agni swept down and scooped up Śiva's divine seed in his beak and carried it off. It was so powerful that it began to burn him and even he, the god of fire could hardly stand the heat. Down below, the mighty river Ganges offered to carry it for him, and so he dropped Śiva's seed into her rushing torrent. After some time, it proved too hot even for the mighty river, and as her surface started to steam, Gaṅgā deposited it along her banks in a marshland, safe from harm. As soon as Śiva's seed met the earth, a radiant child was spawned.

So radiant was this son of Śiva that he caught the eye of the six goddesses of the constellation Kṛttikā, who then immediately descended to tend to his needs. Since each were eager to nurse him, Śiva's son manifested 6 heads so that they may all nurse him at the same time. Nursed by the Kṛttikā Goddesses, this son of Śiva was named Kārttikeya. He soon grew strong and powerful and was appointed Commander of the Celestial Army. The gods delighted as Kārttikeya mounted a campaign to retake the throne of heaven, and destroy the demonic Taraka.

Kārttikeya has many names, including Kumāra, Murugan, Subramanya, and Skanda, after which Skandāsana is named. This pose strengthens your core. It demands balance, poise, and focus—qualities required of great warriors. Take note also that warriors are grounded, respectful, and centered. True warriors always have their heart in it, valuing and believing in what they're fighting for.

MOUNTAIN POSE
TĀḌĀSANA

ŚIVA'S MOUNTAIN ABODE

THEMES
Foundation
Attention
Grounding

EONS AGO THERE WAS A GREAT DROUGHT upon the earth. Water is the essence of life; drought brings death and destruction. And so, the creatures were parched, the plant life was wilted, and the humans were miserable. Concerned for the suffering creatures of the globe, the earth goddess, Pṛthvī, cried out to the heavens. Lord Viṣṇu, the sustainer and keeper of the world, heard her cry and immediately set out to find a solution to this dire problem. Uncertain as to the course of action to be taken, Viṣṇu set out to the abode of Brahmā, creator of the universe, who would surely know what to do. Upon arrival, a booming voice proclaimed, "Welcome, Lord Viṣṇu!" Before him, upon his celestial lotus sat Lord Brahmā himself, shining, wizened, with silky gray hair falling from all four of his heads. "I've been expecting you," said Lord Brahmā.

Lord Viṣṇu bowed reverently and proceeded without delay to convey the dire state of things, beseeching him, "We must not let the earth realm perish! It is there that all beings work out their karmas. We must do something, but I do not know what. Surely, you have something in mind, Grandfather, having created Earth and the cosmos?"

"Well, it seems to me that in times of drought," Brahmā calmly responded, variously stroking his four beards, "the solution can only be one thing—water."

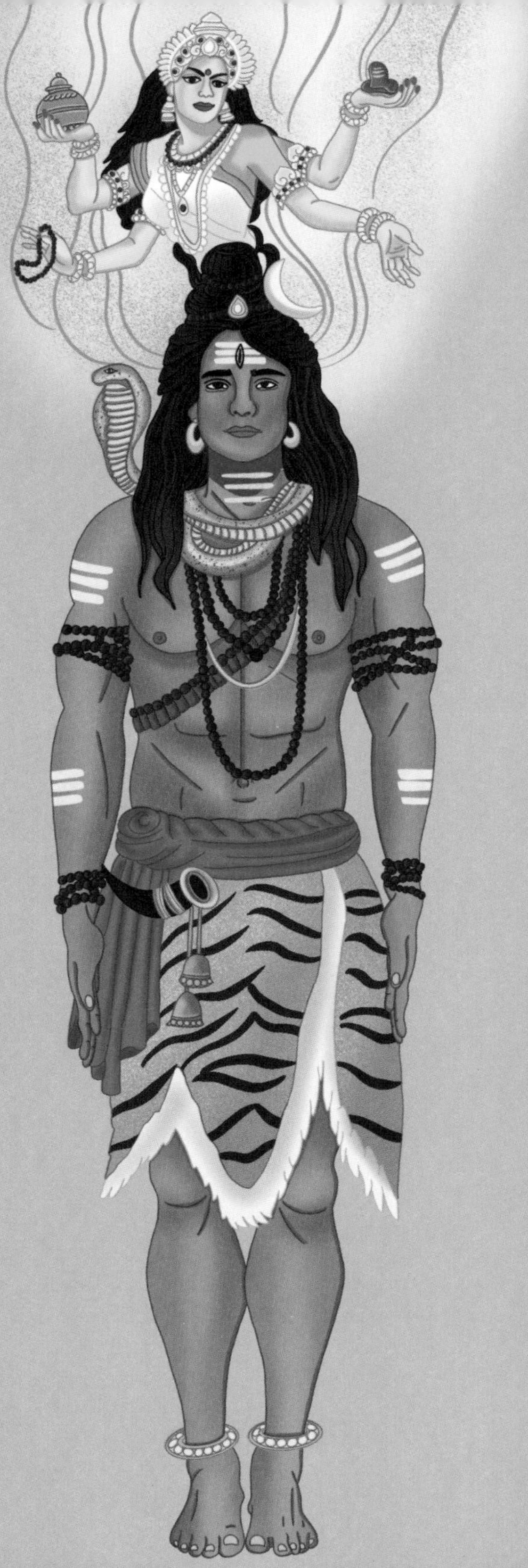

"But Lord Brahmā, there is no water to be found on the earth!"

"Well then, you had better divert some water from elsewhere, hadn't you?"

"Elsewhere?" responded Viṣṇu, perplexed, and becoming increasingly exasperated.

"There are many realms and many sorts of beings in this glorious creation of mine! Go seek out the great celestial river, Gaṅgā, and ask her to descend to the earth. She should serve as the solution to all of your problems." With that, Brahmā returned to his meditation and Viṣṇu left to seek the realm of Gaṅgā.

Viṣṇu came to the impressive abode of Gaṅgā, and was received by her. But upon being presented with Brahmā's plan, Gaṅgā laughed haughtily and replied, "Earth! Down there? You expect me to vacate the heavens and descend to such realms? Even if I desired to descend, my power is too great. My descent would crack the face of the dried and brittle earth in two. No, this will never do!" Dejected, Viṣṇu took leave of Gaṅgā and returned to Brahmā.

"Back so soon, Lord Viṣṇu?" said Brahmā. Viṣṇu explained his situation and begged again for Brahmā to help. Brahmā scratched his celestial heads, and muttered aloud, "The great Gaṅgā may indeed break the earth, yes. Hmm." Then, stirring from his pensiveness, he looked up at Viṣṇu and said, "I do not yet know the answer to this dilemma, but my intuition tells me that you must seek out the mighty Śiva—he will know how to proceed." Viṣṇu thanked Grandfather Brahmā and set out with haste for the abode of Śiva.

Viṣṇu arrived upon the very heights of the earth plane, in the Himālayan mountains, into the powerful meditative presence of the great yogī, Śiva. Clothed in animal skin, his body coated with sacred ash, Śiva graciously interrupted his cosmic trance and half-opened his celestial eyes, sensing Viṣṇu's arrival.

"Praise be to Śiva, Lord of Yogīs!" proclaimed Viṣṇu, bowing.

"Hail, Viṣṇu, Protector of the earth!" replied Viṣṇu, returning his reverence. The ever watchful third eye of Śiva had witnessed Viṣṇu's plight unfolding and, needing no explanation, he spoke:

"Return to Gaṅgā and inform her that I request her presence here in my Himālayan abode. Tell her that I await her descent. I will take care of the rest," and returned to his meditation. Fully trusting that Śiva would handle situation, Viṣṇu respectfully took leave of the lord and returned to the abode of Gaṅgā to deliver Śiva's message.

"Lord Śiva has asked me to descend?" asked Gaṅgā, astonished. "Surely, I cannot refuse the Destroyer!" she mused aloud. "But what of the earth? How will she bear my might? Still, if Śiva says descend, then I shall, and leave it to you to piece together her remains."

Prideful as ever, but wise enough to comply with the request of Śiva himself, Gaṅgā flung herself from the Heavens, downwards to the earthly plane, flowing directly toward the abode of Śiva, certain, though she was, that she would crack the earth in two. Śiva positioned himself so as to receive the turbulent might of Gaṅgā upon his own head. Thus, as she descended, the celestial river found herself slowed, calmed, and grounded by the yogic presence of the lord. Time slowed down, as though all space were converging upon his head. In his intoxicating presence, Gaṅgā experienced herself as no more than a single drop of dew amid his matted locks. She lingered for an eternal moment in his expansiveness before, inebriated, she slid down his body, paying homage and loving respect to his feet, before continuing down the Himālayas to hydrate and bless the earth. Pacified by the grounding power of Śiva, the Ganges descended to Earth where she nourishes and purifies countless souls to this day, all by the grounding grace of Śiva.

There are two types of standing: mindless standing, and standing with attention. By default, many of us simply mill about, standing here and there to pass the time. The soldier stands to attention, with attention, and all the more so, the yogī. Like a tree whose roots burrow down toward the center of the earth, so, too, does the yogī plant their feet firmly on the floor in standing tāḍāsana. Beyond the planting of the feet to mirror the roots of the tree, the yogī in tāḍāsana mirrors the trunk, as their body is erect, allowing the flow of life sap to vertically permeate their being, aligned with the spine. Just as the branches of the tree reach out to touch the sky, so, too, does the yogī in tāḍāsana elongate their body, the top of their head touching the sky as it were, collapsing the space between heaven and earth. This energized, attentive standing is more than milling about, it is the standing which we refer to when something stands the test of time. This is the standing of trees, of pyramids, of mountains. Śiva, Lord of Yogīs, both symbolizes and inhabits the mountains. Like Śiva, the mountains are grounded, secure, enduring, majestic. He is the yang principle to support the yin of śakti. He is the riverbed without which the river could not flow.

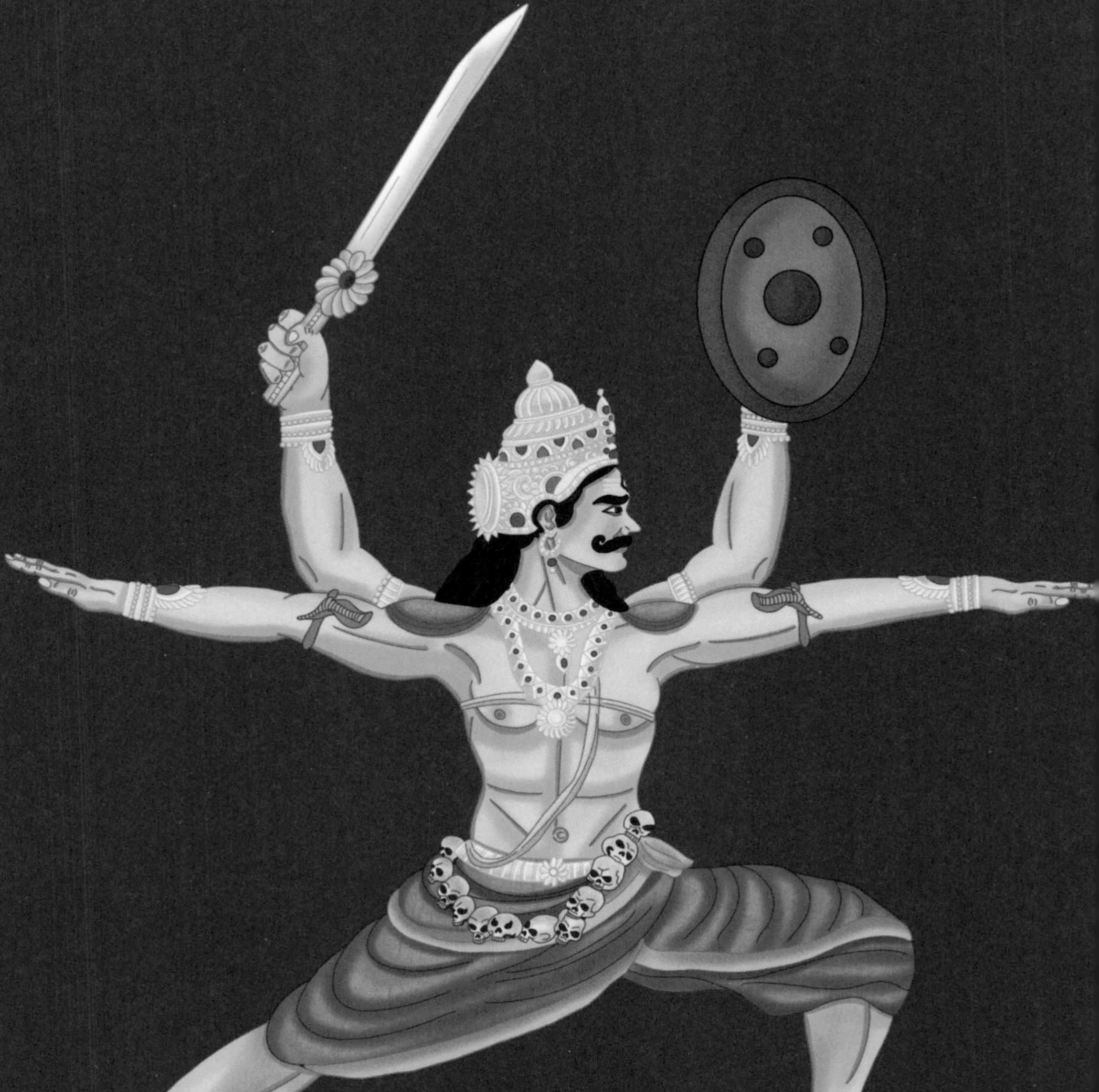

WARRIOR POSE
VĪRABHADRĀSANA

ŚIVA'S COMPOSED WRATH

THEMES
Power
Poise
Assertion

SINCE THE DAWN OF THIS WORLD, the dance of dualities pulling this way and that has propelled existence ever onwards. Śiva and Śakti are these very opposites; cosmic soulmates, destined to be brought together and flung apart, again and again throughout the many different incarnations of Śakti. Perhaps the most tragic and beautiful of all these unions is to be found in the story of Śiva and Satī.

Śakti, the mother of name and form, the very fabric of this universe, has assumed many manifestations in her timeless embrace of Śiva. Perhaps none of these were so loving and pure as Satī. Satī longed deeply for Śiva, thought only of him, and invoked his mantras every day; her heart was truly devoted to him, and she knew they were destined for one another.

Satī, however, was the daughter of proud Dakṣa, son of Lord Brahmā. When the time had come for his fair daughter to be wed, he threw a grand party, inviting many a suitor of high breeding. Though Satī's heart beat only for Śiva, she knew her father would never approve. For how could anyone of repute accept as a son-in-law, an unkept, unwashed yogī with matted locks, clad in little more than a tiger-skin loincloth and the ceremonial ash that covered his flesh? Fated though their love may be, Satī knew that it could never be simple.

It was the custom during such times, that the bride-to-be select her chosen groom by adorning him with a garland of roses (much to the chagrin of the rejected suitors). So, from the balcony of her father's mansion, Satī tossed the garland into the air, so high that none could begin to plot the trajectory of its descent. All were breathless as the garland began to descend upon the congregation of eager bachelors. But as it fell, Satī quietly whispered a mantra to Śiva, summoning him to her with the sincerity of her heart. He appeared among the crowd, perfectly placed to be adorned by the falling garland. Satī was delighted. Śiva, too, was overjoyed, and though Dakṣa was outraged, he knew that the fate of his daughter was bound by the garland. She had tricked him, and he had no choice but to begrudgingly accept Śiva into his family. So, the two were wed, and were quite happy together. Satī gladly gave up her glamorous life as the daughter of Dakṣa to live in Śiva's mountain shack. Their days passed in the ecstasy of cosmic union and their souls became ever more deeply entwined.

But Dakṣa's resentment festered, and he could not forgive his daughter's betrayal. She had humiliated him, and in his bitterness, he sought retribution. He held an important event—a grand fire sacrifice. He invited everyone of significance, including his daughter, but not his own son-in-law, Śiva. All of the gods and celestial beings would enjoy a share of the sacrifice, but not him. Satī arrived at the ceremony, infuriated by her father's insult, and demanded an explanation. Dakṣa remained resolute in his pride, and smugly stated that he could invite whomever he wished to his own events. Every fiber of Satī's being was devoted to Śiva, and she could not bear such a slight upon him. In her rage, she lost control, threw herself upon the sacrificial flames, and was consumed by them.

Śiva immediately felt a disturbance. He turned his attention inwards and saw with his yogic vision what had happened. A furious outrage gripped him, and he burned with wrath and contempt toward Dakṣa. With what little composure remained to him, he ripped a piece of his matted locks from his steaming skull and threw it on the ground, uttering a mantra. Where it fell, there appeared before him the great warrior, Vīrabhadra. Though he was spawned of Śiva's wrath and possessed all his power, Vīrabhadra himself retained full emotional control. But driven to action by Śiva's intention, he nonetheless descended upon Dakṣa's sacrifice and wrought havoc upon it. None could withstand him. Dakṣa paid the price for his pride and ignorance, and was decapitated by the fearsome warrior.

Soon after Vīrabhadra's grisly deed was done, Śiva's anger gave way to anguish, and he wept for his lost soulmate. Softened by grief, he came to the scene of the sacrifice, and taking pity on Dakṣa, replaced his head with that of a goat and resurrected him. Once revived, Dakṣa immediately realized the ignorance of his ways, and asked Śiva for forgiveness. Together, they grieved the loss of Satī. But Śiva was ultimately inconsolable. He took up the charred body of his beloved and, maddened by loss, carried her on his shoulder as he wandered, heartbroken, throughout the cosmos, until compassionate Viṣṇu intervened with a proposal: Satī's sacred corpse would be disintegrated and dispersed across the land, and each spot where a remnant of Satī landed would become a site of sacred power—a śakti pīṭha—where devotees of the goddess could worship her until the end of days. Śiva agreed, and accepted the wondrous memorialization of his beloved Satī.

Fifty-two such sites of power remain to this day, spread across India, where great temples are built in Satī's honor. The goddess Śakti eventually took the form of Pārvatī and became Śiva's divine lover once again. Śiva never forgot the lesson he learnt about the need to reign in his wrath. Dakṣa, too, learned the value of humility. And the great warrior Vīrabhadra remains on guard even now, posed to oppose ignorance. When you stand in warrior pose, take the opportunity to compose yourself and gather your strength, ready to face whatever situations may arise. The story of Vīrabhadra can give us the courage to take swift and decisive action to combat whatever ignorance we may encounter, within as well as without.

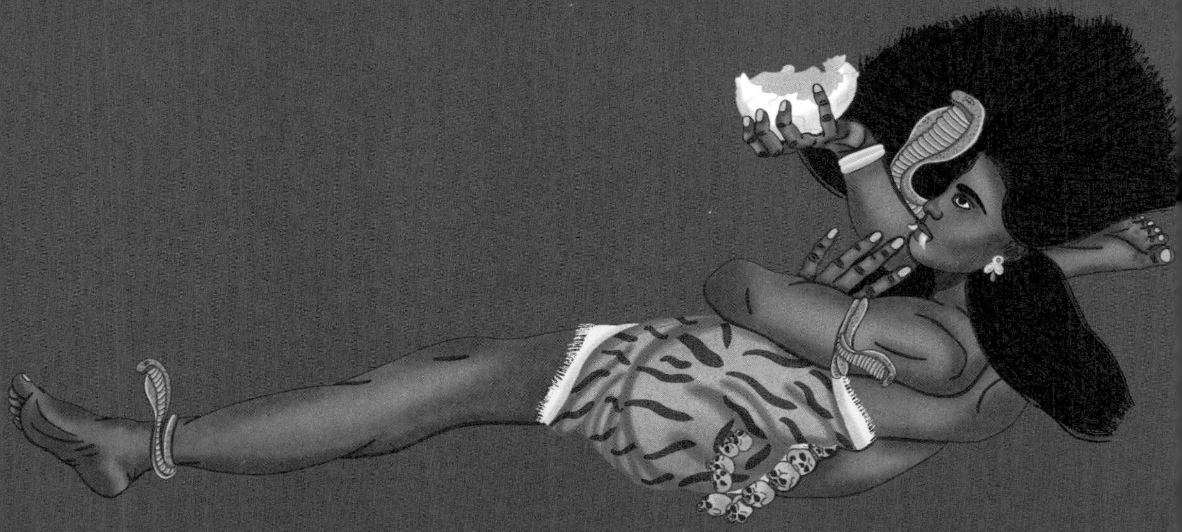

TERROR POSE
BHAIRAVĀSANA

BHAIRAVA,
ŚIVA'S WRATH

THEMES
Courage
Humility
Purification

THERE ARE THREE VERY IMPORTANT cosmic functions to be fullfilled in the universe: creation, preservation, and destruction. These functions are carried out by the three gods, Brahmā the Creator, Viṣṇu the Preserver, and Śiva the Destroyer. This trinity of divinities is known as the *trimūrti*. But which one of these divinities is the greatest of all? Which of their functions is the most important? This very question was, in fact, entertained by the gods themselves one day:

"Surely, as the creator of all things, I am the greatest of all," said Lord Brahmā. Were it not for me, nothing at all would exist. Therefore, it cannot be doubted that I wield the greatest of cosmic powers!"

"So it is, Lord Brahmā. You are the creator of all things," replied Viṣṇu, "but once you have withdrawn from creation and retired to your meditation, it is I who must ensure the universe's upkeep, preserving it, eon after eon. I am forever incarnating in this or that form, just to prevent events on the earth plane from spiraling out of control! Without my tortoise incarnation, the demons and gods never would have procured the Elixir of Immortality, and without my incarnation as Kṛṣṇa, the great Mahābhārata war could not have been won, and evil would have prevailed upon the earth. Therefore, my cosmic role as Preserver is clearly greater than yours, Lord Brahmā."

Then Śiva the Destroyer, Lord of all Yogīs spoke: "Creation and preservation do indeed both require great power, my lords. Yet consider that once you, Brahmā, have created the universe and withdrawn from it, and while you, Viṣṇu, toil to maintain it, I engage in meditation and, for as long as the universe persists, amass extraordinary yogic power. With this power, I shall annihilate the cosmos at the end of time. All your creations will expire, and all attempts at preservation will ultimately fail. I surely possess more power than the cosmos itself, for how else could I be capable of destroying it? At the end of the age, I alone will remain. So it must be, in order for Brahmā to be born anew at the dawn of the next. Truly, there can be no question of which one of us wields more power."

Viṣṇu was humbled, and recognizing the greatness of Śiva, he contentedly conceded: "It stands to reason that you do indeed wield the greatest power; the power to annihilate all things, garnered through your extraordinary yogic practice. Hail Śiva, Lord of Yogīs!"

But Brahmā was proud of his creation, and he grew agitated by Śiva's words. "Do neither of you realize that I am Grandfather of all Creation? What would exist without my creative power? Śiva, you think you are powerful, but without me, you are nought but an unwashed, reclusive, self-absorbed ascetic! We may each have five heads, but my divine eyes see clearly, while yours appear clouded with ceremonial ash!"

Viṣṇu gasped. He would not dare to insult Śiva in such a manner, knowing full well the danger that Śiva's terrible anger could pose. But boastful Brahmā had kindled the Destroyer's wrath. The cosmos quaked and grew black as ink as Śiva's fury grew. Śiva himself grew dark and scowled. He tore a shred from his fingernail and tossed it on to the earth, as he uttered an ominous mantra. From that fingernail grew a fearsome warrior named Bhairava (also known as Kāla-Bhairava), an embodiment of Śiva's supreme wrath. Bhairava's bare, indigo skin proclaimed his intensity and strength. Fearsome fangs protruded from his face. One of his four hands was empty, but in the others, he carried a scythe, a trident, and a noose.

Before Brahmā could utter another insolent word, Bhairava, ablaze with Śiva's outrage, lunged with terrifying speed, and severed the fifth head of Brahmā, which had uttered the insult. Bhairava carries Brahmā's decapitated skull in his fourth hand to this day. Upon decapitation, the Creator immediately realized the error of his arrogance.

Humbled by the ordeal, and purified by Śiva's punishment, Brahmā recognized the supremacy of Śiva's colossal power. He exclaimed with all four of his remaining heads, facing in all directions, "Glory to Śiva, Great Destroyer! Hail Śiva, Great God, Lord of Yogīs! Victory to Bhairava, Śiva's Fearsome Wrath!"

Bhairava represents the most formidable, destructive aspect of Śiva. He is fearless, and fearsome. He represents the courage and force required to combat toxic ego, whether within or without. The arrogance to be found in the Creator mirrors that found throughout his creation. This egoic aspect, found in self and others, thwarts divine aspirations and curtails divine consciousness. It must be combatted for yogic power to be recognized and realized. It is the ego that sees destruction as an ending, as a negative thing. The soul sees destruction of material obstructions as the great spiritual blessing it is, a blessing bestowed by Śiva.

We feel the power of divine decapitation in Bhairavāsana, as we submit our own heads in this pose. It reminds us of Brahmā's arrogance and subsequent humility—his transformation from the darkness of ego to the light of divine consciousness. Once decapitated, Brahmā is purified of toxic, blinding ego, and rid of attachments and obstructions to the realization of divinity. Strive to remember this tale, and realize its wisdom, when you assume Bhairavāsana.

DOG POSE
ŚVĀNĀSANA

BHAIRAVA'S CANINE VEHICLE

THEMES
Loyalty
Ferocity
Power

Several Hindu deities have vāhanas—animal vehicles. Viṣṇu's vehicle is the eagle Garuḍa, Durgā's is the lion, and Gaṇeśa's is the mouse. These vehicles are a key component of the symbolism of the deity and provide insight into their energy. In most cases, the significance of the deity's vehicle is quite intuitive. For example, the poised, powerful, regal Durgā rides the lion, the king of the jungle, into battle.

In some cases, the vehicle doesn't represent the energy of the deity, but the energy to be transformed by the deity. The best example of this is Gaṇeśa presiding over the mouse. The great elephant-headed god is the lord of wisdom, grounding, and auspicious beginnings. He represents the part of self that the ancients called the *buddhi*, the truth recognizing intellect. In order to hear our voice of inner wisdom, we must silence the chatter of the mind—that is—the part of the self which processes sensation, impulse, habit, and emotion, that the ancients call the *manas*. This is represented by Gaṇeśa's vehicle, the mouse. Wisdom can ground and settle the mind; though it may be full of fear, scurrying to –and fro, the grounding energy of Gaṇeśa can bring stillness, poise, and access to higher cognitive functions.

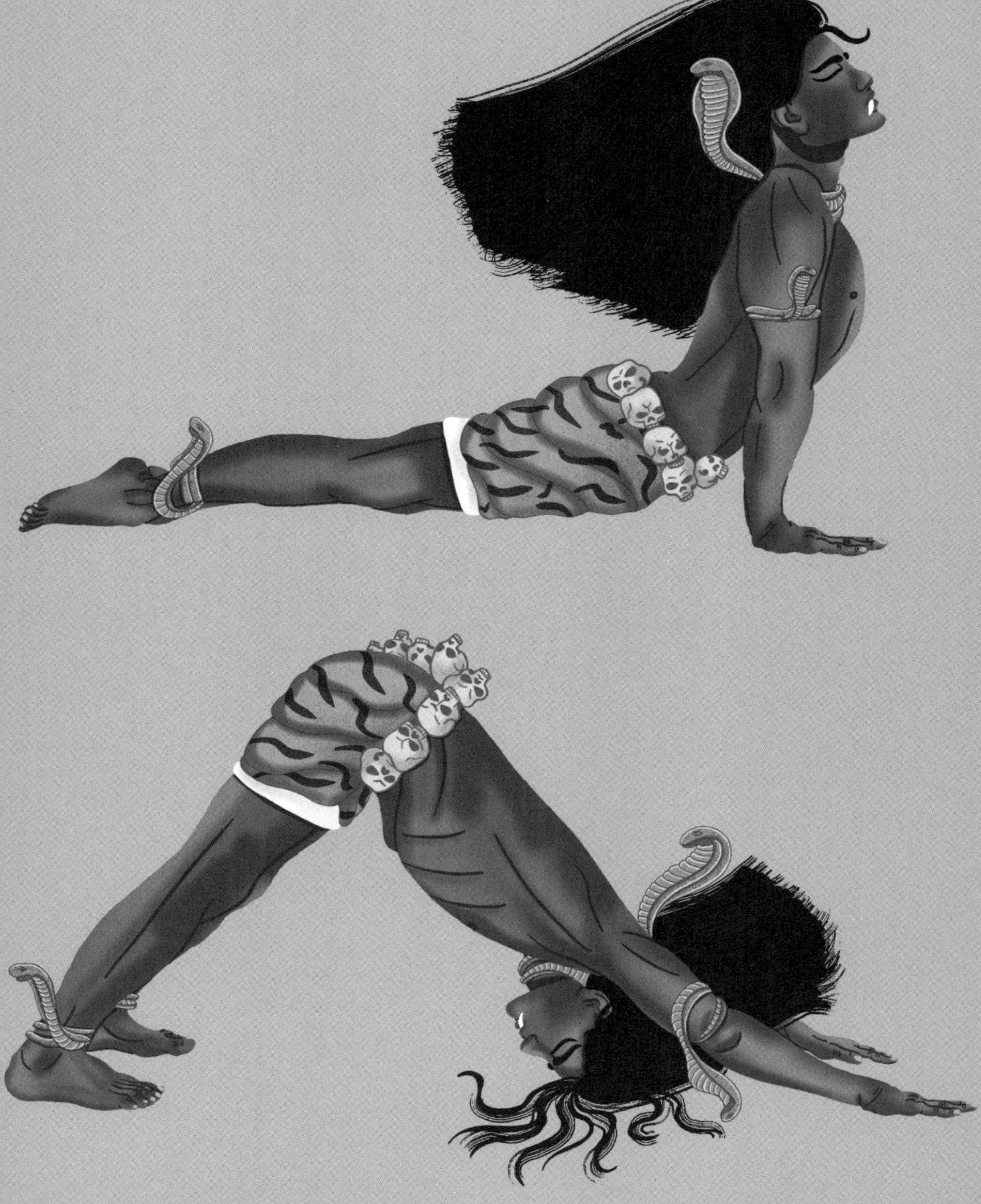

Bhairava's vehicle is the dog (śvāna). The dog brings with it a wide range of connotations. Within the realm of Indian mythology, we have Saramā, the female dog from the Ṛg Veda belonging to the pantheon of gods, along with Death's (Yama's) four-eyed dogs guarding the gates of hell. The vehicle of Bhairava, who reprents, Śiva's divine wrath, teaches us about his energy. Due to associations created by our own modern, Western conditioning, we may well see the dog as a faithful and loving companion to human beings. But let's try and think outside of the box of our conditioning, and understand the essence of canine energy. Think of a time and space before the domestication of canines. Call to mind the wild natures of the fox and the wolf, the jackal and the cayote. Like Bhairava, these canine creatures are fierce and formidable creatures—sleek, striking, and dangerous carnivores, skilled at the hunt. They may well lunge at their prey in an instant, aiming for the jugular. So canines, much like Bhairava, can be quite terrifying creatures.

Canines can indeed be ferocious, but they also live and hunt with great intelligence, and with purpose. Once you are able to form a bond with them, they are loyal and protective. The ferocity with which a canine hunts is the same ferocity with which it protects. Just as one might invoke Bhairava for protection, so too, might one employ the service of a powerful, formidable guard dog. It's a question of transforming that raw, wild power into a protective energy. The dog can be domesticated, and so too can the wild energy of Śiva and even that of his wrath, Bhairava. Like the dog, spiritual power is wild and dangerous, but with the correct training and guidance, it can be harnessed to power spiritual growth.

Beyond being powerful and fearsome, the dog in the Indic context has been regarded as polluting, eating scraps, and sifting through garbage. One must realize that the vast majority of dogs in the Indic subcontinent do not live in human homes, but have a society of their own at the margins of human affairs. Just as the dog in this context brings with it associations of pollution and marginality, so too does Bhairava. In fact, in addition to being a mainstream Hindu deity, he is the presiding deity of the holy city Benaras where countless Hindus cremate their dead and scatter their ashes in the Ganges. Bhairava represents the tantric transformation that takes elements of marginality, transgression, and pollution and transmutes them for spiritual growth.

There is a famous story near the end of the great Sanskrit epic, Mahābhārata, where the royal hero Yudhiṣṭhira allows a dog to accompany him to the gates of heaven. The gods object to so "polluting" the divine realms with its presence, denying the dog entry into heaven. But Yudhiṣṭhira was taken by the loyalty of the dog, and returned his loyalty by declaring to the gods of heaven that he would not leave the dog behind. As it turned out, the dog was Yudhiṣṭhira's father, Dharma, the god of virtue, in disguise—he had been testing Yudhiṣṭhira's virtue all along. Here we see the dual aspect of the canine spirit: The purest of hearts even in the most unclean of bodies.

Just as canines have both wild and tame personas, so there are two versions of Dog Pose. Upwards facing dog has to do with working with the wild canine energy. This is a heating pose that activates the upward flow of kuṇḍalinī. The head is above the heart, extending to the heavens. Downward Dog, on the other hand, is a cooling pose. It offers the grounding presence and companionship of a domesticated dog. Śiva is sometimes called Paśupati, Lord of Beasts, because his refined consciousness is said to be able to effortlessly tame wild beasts. In downward dog, the head is below the heart, grounding into the earth. Hands and feet are firmly planted on the floor. In this pose, we allow our wild energies to be calmed, like a tame and loving dog. In these two poses we see the range of expression we can find in canine creatures. By understanding the mythology of Bhairava we understand the transformative power of that energy in the life of the yogī.

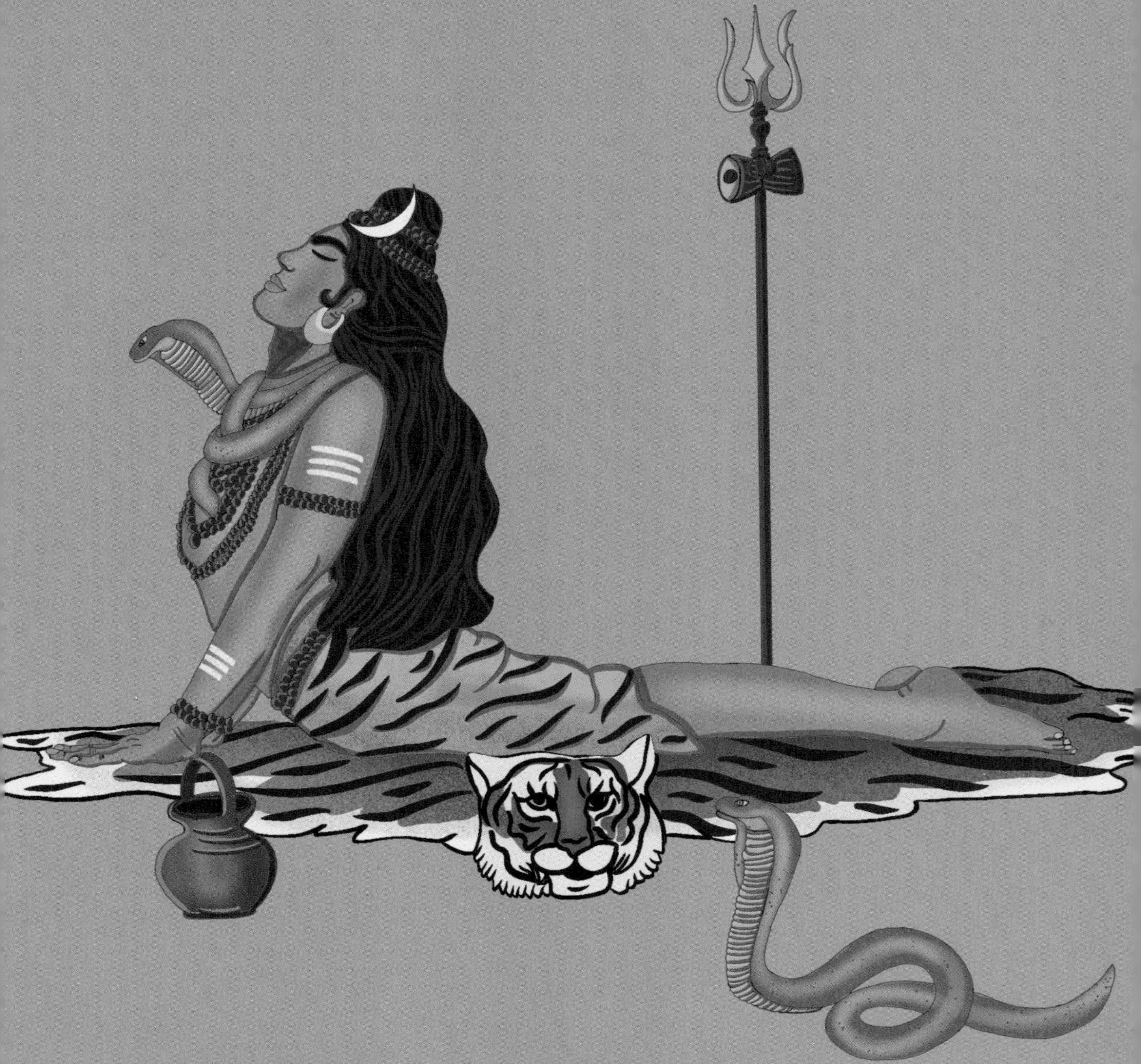

COBRA POSE
BHUJĀṄGĀSANA

THE CHURNING OF THE COSMIC OCEAN (PART II)

THEMES
Power
Persistence
Neutralization

IN THE EARLY DAYS OF THE UNIVERSE, the Devas (gods) and Daityas (demons) agreed to put aside their age-old feud and work together to find the Elixir of Immortality. To find it, they first had to churn the cosmic ocean, the Milky Way itself. For their churning pole, they chose the great Mount Mandara, and for their churning rope, Vāsuki, king of the serpents, had volunteered his body. Viṣṇu, the Preserver, had transformed himself into a tortoise upon whose shell Mount Mandara could be placed, at the bottom of the ocean. Vāsuki wrapped his body around the Mountain, and with the Devas and Daityas each taking hold of him on either side, the churning began.

Like all worthwhile endeavors, the churning was, at first, arduous. The ocean was as dense and thick as an unploughed field in the wilderness. It scarcely relented to their toiling. Without warning, and after only a handful of heaves to-and-fro, the ocean emitted a vile indigo colored poison high into the heavens above! Both Devas and Daityas gasped as the crude substance launched into the air and began to descend upon them. What an ironic fate to be destroyed by deadly poison while in search of immortal life!

All eyes were on the poison, including the third eye of Lord Śiva, the Destroyer, who watched from afar, in deep yogic trance in his abode on Mount Kailāśa. He interrupted his meditation and swiftly disembarked. Knowing that no being could withstand the potency of the oceanic toxins, he graced the scene, opened his mouth, and allowed the poison to enter it. The Daityas and Devas reeled with both relief and alarm. Would the great Śiva sacrifice himself in order to save the universe? What dreadful fate would ensue for the universe if he were destroyed? All present knew of Śiva's cosmic role. At the end of each age, he performed his dance of transcendental bliss, destroying the universe, so that Brahmā may create it anew. Countless creations have thus issued forth, but without the Destroyer, there could be no subsequent creation!

All eyes looked on in awe as the poison entered the mouth of Lord Śiva. To their surprise, he did not swallow it. All were perplexed by the fact that he also did not spit it out. Rather, he lodged the cosmic venom in his divine throat and, with his ascetic power, neutralized it. His throat turned deep blue, and from that day onwards Śiva was given the name of Nīlakaṇṭha, "He whose throat is blue." "Glory to Śiva!" praised the entourage of demons, gods, and other celestial beings. "Glory to Mahādeva, the Great God! Glory to the Lord of the Yogīs! Glory to the Blue-Throated One!" Thus it was that the great Lord Śiva fullfilled his divine role in the Churning of the Ocean.

Having been purified of its dreadful poisons like a mind freed of toxic perceptions, or like a heart unburdened by malignant emotion, the ocean began to flow more freely, cooperating with the forces acting upon it. Like the ocean of our consciousness, it started off crude, and required enormous "churning" via introspection, meditation, and therapeutic processes to become refined. And so, with each swivel of Mount Mandara, with each thrust of the arms of the demons and gods, the ocean became more refined and more amenable to the quest for immortality. As it was continually churned, the ocean offered up its finest riches, each more rarified than the last, and all of which were distributed among the Daityas and Devas.

Though sweat pervaded their weary brows and they gasped for breath, they did not abandon their cause. They were intent on procuring the elixir of everlasting life. So great was their effort, and so refined became the ocean, that it bestowed upon them a resplendent orb of cool delight; the moon itself was born. Because of his colossal feat, the moon was offered at the feet of Lord Śiva who embraced it, and donned it amid his matted locks. So captivating was the radiance of this sight that the entire celestial assembly paused for a moment to admire the newly born moon.

The cobra adorns Śiva as his sacred garland. His blue throat is a symbol of auspiciousness and power, showing that while power can be dangerous, it need not be malevolent. The cobra is also a symbol of rising kuṇḍalinī śakti; the divine energy that travels up the subtle spine. Once it reaches the crown, one is awakened. The cobra's ability to stand up tall, unique among snake species, represents the unique capacity of the human spine to occupy a fully upright posture. When the kuṇḍalinī energy at the base of the spine is awoken during spiritual practice, it dredges up the poisonous crud we need to address. Upon consistent growth, the śakti yields riches, each more refined than the last.

We mortals have much to learn from the power of Lord Śiva. If we fail to learn the lesson of Śiva, we will either swallow (internalize) or spit out (externalize) the toxins of our experiences. What kind of state would we enjoy if we were able to damage neither self nor other with the toxicity of our suffering? What kind of state might our world enjoy if it remained unsullied by venom? Śiva is a potent example of neutralizing the poison of life, thus safeguarding the welfare of self and others.

This story is continued on page 99.

LORD OF DANCE POSE
TĀṆḌAVĀSANA

ŚIVA'S COSMIC DANCE OF BLISS

THEMES
Grounding
Balance
Energy

THOUSANDS OF YEARS FROM NOW, this age will end, but if we pay close attention, we may notice that endings are illusions. The seeming ending of one thing always marks the commencement of another. Nothing comes from nothing, and nothing passes into nothing. The process of transformation from one thing to another is all that exists.

Time creates all things, only to devour them again, that they may be recreated. The dissolution of this age will give rise to a new creation as the universe continues to cycle through creation, destruction and re-creation. Nevertheless, at the end of this age, something colossal will occur: Śiva will rise from his cosmic meditation, assume his Lord of Dance form and perform his dance of bliss to annihilate all things. This dance will dissolve everything into the same primordial ocean of potential that it emerged from at the dawn of creation, just as he has countless times before, and just as he will, at the close of countless universes to come.

Upon the mountains, high above the world, away from the social order, soon to be dissolved, Śiva's matted locks will sway in rhythm as he beats his drum in wild, shamanic fervor. The structures of society, like wheels within wheels, come and go, arise and dissolve, in the course of ordinary time. But at the end of the age, all will be ripe for its own complete destruction; devoured by the endless march of

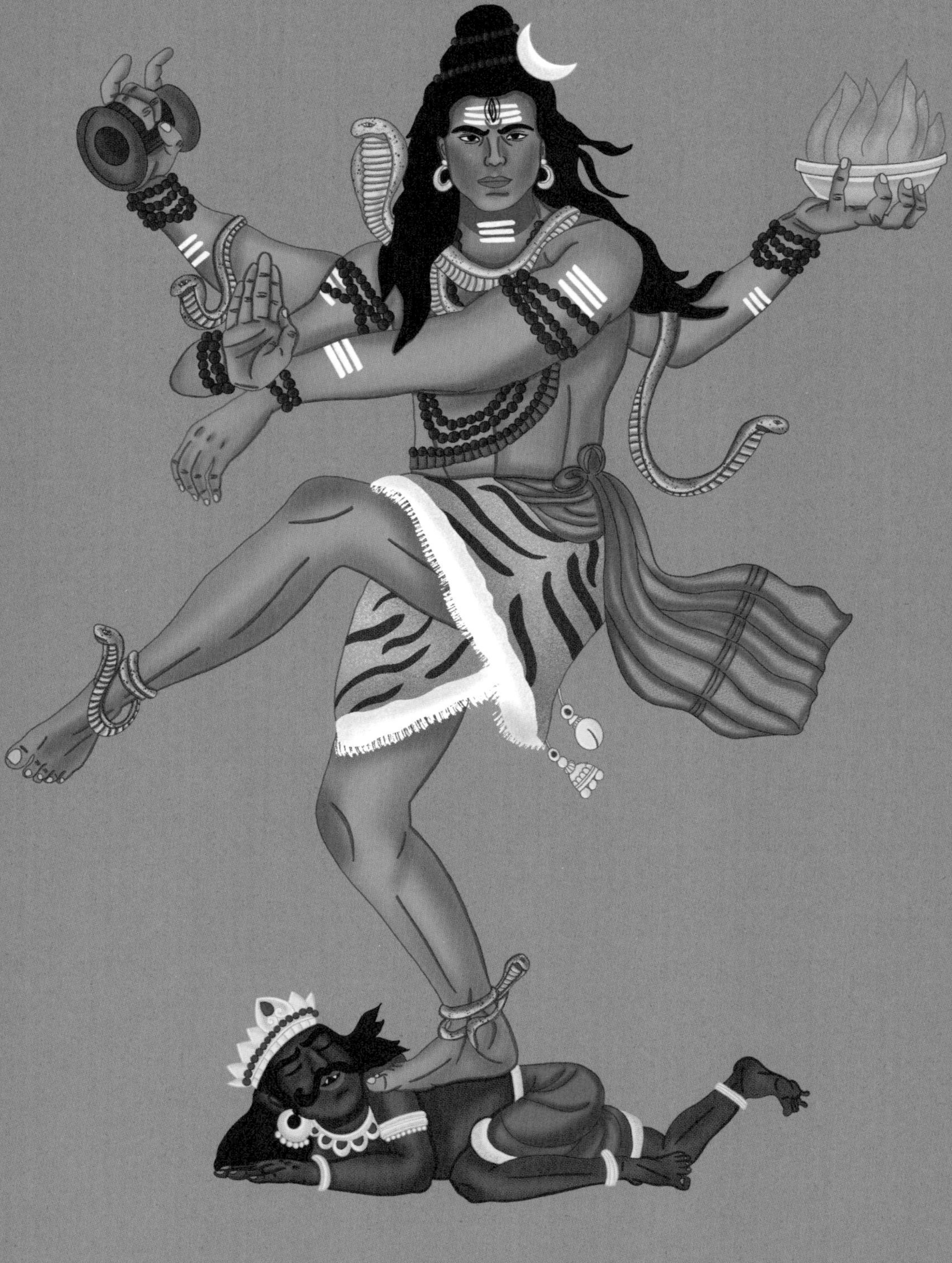

cosmic time; returned to its original formlessness beyond all forms by Śiva's dance of transcendence.

Through his dance, being and becoming will finally be fully united. The moon, residing as she does amid his matted locks, will spin and flail about with him; her femininity grounded by his masculine energy. Śiva and Śakti will, at last, merge in fullness. Śakti, whose power underpins all becoming, will withdraw from creation, allowing for its dissolution. She will recede from the universe and become the very dance itself. Śiva and Śakti will become inseparable, the masculine indistinguishable from the feminine; the dancer indistinguishable from the dance. The flames of transformation will fall down around them, encircling them as their ecstasy initiates the apocalypse. The phenomenal world, everything from the atomic to the galactic, will be dissolved in Śiva's blissful dance.

Śiva's Lord of Dance pose assumes four arms. In the back right hand, he holds the drum which beats out the rise and fall of all things in time. His drum represents the heartbeat of creation, and brings about the circulation of our experience. Despite the deafening pulse of his drum, his front right hand assumes the "fear-not" gesture (abhaya mudra) bestowing blessings upon the world. His right leg stands on the dwarf of ignorance, who represents separation, attachment, confusion; those who take as real the decaying and illusory world, soon to be dissolved. Yet Śiva's graceful, active left foot represents the blessing of revelation of all beyond māyā, beyond illusion, and the emancipation of enlightenment which accompanies it. This is the energy present in Śiva's "Death-Conquering" mantra:

> tryambakaṁ yajāmahe sugandhiṁ puṣṭi-vardhanaṁ
> urvārukam iva bandhanān mṛtyor mukṣīya māmṛtāt
>
> *Ṛg Veda VII.59.12*

> We worship the three-eyed one, who is fragrant and who nourishes all beings. As is the ripened cucumber freed from its bondage (to the vine), may He liberate us from death for the sake of immortality.

As his front right hand gestures "fear not," so his front left hand points the way to the path of freedom. His back left hand carries with it the fires of transformation, which tear the world asunder. He pierces through the phenomenal world in step with his dance of bliss. He is powerful, and he is perfectly poised. So, too, does the yogī's perception pierce through the mundane, while yet dancing in divine step. As the divine conceals, so the divine reveals.

Remember to ground in the line of energy between heaven and earth. This is how this pose begins. Once grounded, activate Śiva's cosmic dance pose, striking a balance between grounding and grace. In this pose, you can find the elegant order within the chaos of life; a sense of poise among the clamor of the days; the blissful surrender amid the inevitable decaying of all things.

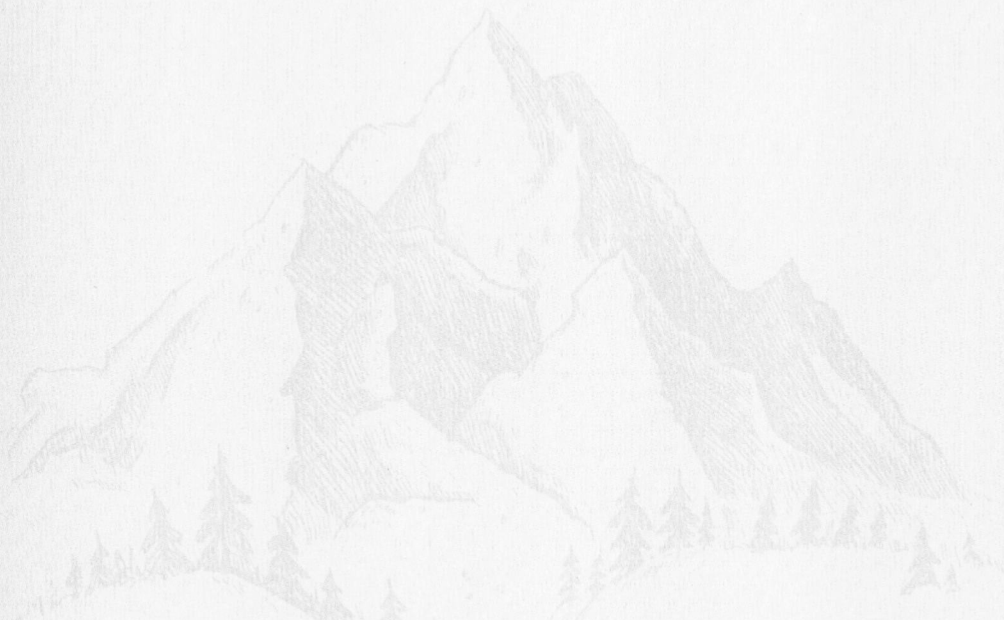

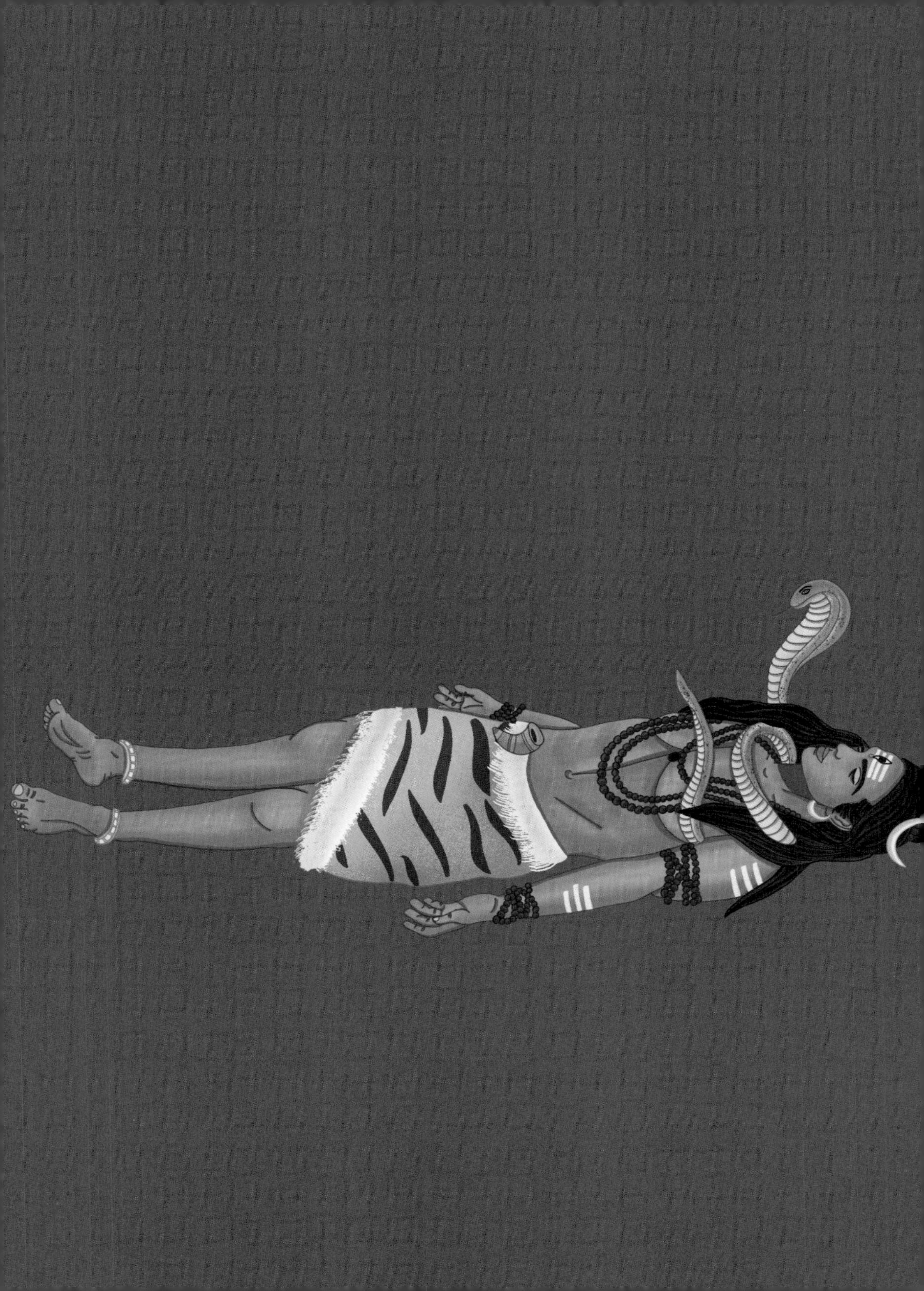

CORPSE POSE
ŚAVĀSANA

ŚIVA AND THE POWER OF INERTIA

THEMES
Bearing witness
Stillness
Inertia

LONG AGO, THE GREAT DEMON TARAKA had taken over heaven and terrorized the gods. Taraka's greatest strength was that he could only be defeated by a child of Śiva, and none were less likely to father a child than he, reclusive and celibate as he was. So, in desperation, Indra and the other gods of heaven decided to send the god of erotic desire, Kāma, to Śiva's mountain abode. His task was to target Śiva with his arrows of desire, that he may fall in love with the earth goddess, Pārvatī, and have a child with her. Like all incarnations of Śakti, Pārvatī loved Śiva and longed always to be with him.

When Kāma arrived, he saw that Śiva was meditating. His eyes were closed, his consciousness one with the divine, and he was unaware of his immediate surroundings in material creation. Kāma saw that Pārvatī, the daughter of the Mountain was close by, walking close to Śiva's shack, just as the gods of heaven had planned. At that moment, Kāma loosed his arrow, and as it struck the lord, his eyes fluttered open and his awareness returned to his physical location. He became aware of the intoxicating presence of the lovely Pārvatī, and was enticed by her radiance. In that moment, Śiva wanted nothing more than to love Pārvatī, and to express his love by becoming one with her, physically, enjoying the pleasures of embodied existence. But a split second later, he returned to his yogic senses and realized that this shift in his consciousness had been caused by Kāma. A wave of spiritual power surged upwards through Śiva. His third eye opened, and from it, a fearsome blast of yogic fire emanated, instantly incinerating Kāma. Kāma was utterly destroyed, but his deed was done. Śiva, the great ascetic, was in love.

He returned his gaze to Pārvatī, and their eyes locked in loving exchange. Eternity seemed to pass between their glances, and the rapture of their union overtook them. But after a time, a deep concern arose in Pārvatī:

"Great Lord, now that Kāma is destroyed, he can no longer kindle desire among beings. They will isolate themselves and die out. Surely this fate cannot come to pass for the beings of the earth."

"Your beauty is matched by wisdom, my love" he replied. "I will resurrect Kāma in spirit so that desire may dwell in the creatures of Earth, that they may propagate and enjoy material existence, though I myself have no use for Kāma."

"Are you certain about that, Lord?" asked Pārvatī. Her mood had shifted, her loving gaze faded, and her manner had become serious. But Śiva continued:

"Of course! I have raised my spiritual power to the point of transcending desire. Do you not realize this?"

Though he did not know it, Śiva had sparked a deep anger within Pārvatī. The light and colour of her complexion drained away as her presence expanded, darkening the very mountains they stood upon. Even the mighty Śiva trembled as her energetic field grew still larger and blacker. Even he fell to the ground in utter submission, for he was no longer in the presence of Pārvatī. Before him instead was Kālī; the feminine energy of all creation, withdrawn from the universe, and manifested in her most great and terrifying form. Śiva lay corpse like, utterly still. Kālī stood over him, and her terrible laughter echoed throughout the cosmos. Then she spoke:

"You are the consciousness of the universe, and I am its energy. Without my power all beings merely lie inert as you do now. I am the primordial power that propels the galaxies, and all being within the cosmos. I am desire, without which there is no action. Even your meditation is born of your desire. How else could it be? You are the walker, I am the walk, you the dancer, and I, the dance. But when my energy is removed from you, you are awareness alone, incapable of all action. Behold, my colossal power as I return it to the universe and all beings within it, including you, Great Lord!"

Śiva learned a great lesson that day about the power of Śakti, the feminine divine, and its relationship to desire. He learned what it's like to be completely inert, and witness creation's dynamic play. When Kālī withdraws from Śiva, he is little more than śava—a corpse. And so, as you embrace the inert stillness of śavāsana, practice witnessing. Cease becoming for that time, and embrace being. Through the practice of divine inertia, of śavāsana, the capacity for witnessing from stillness can come to accompany you, even as you move through the turbulence of daily life.

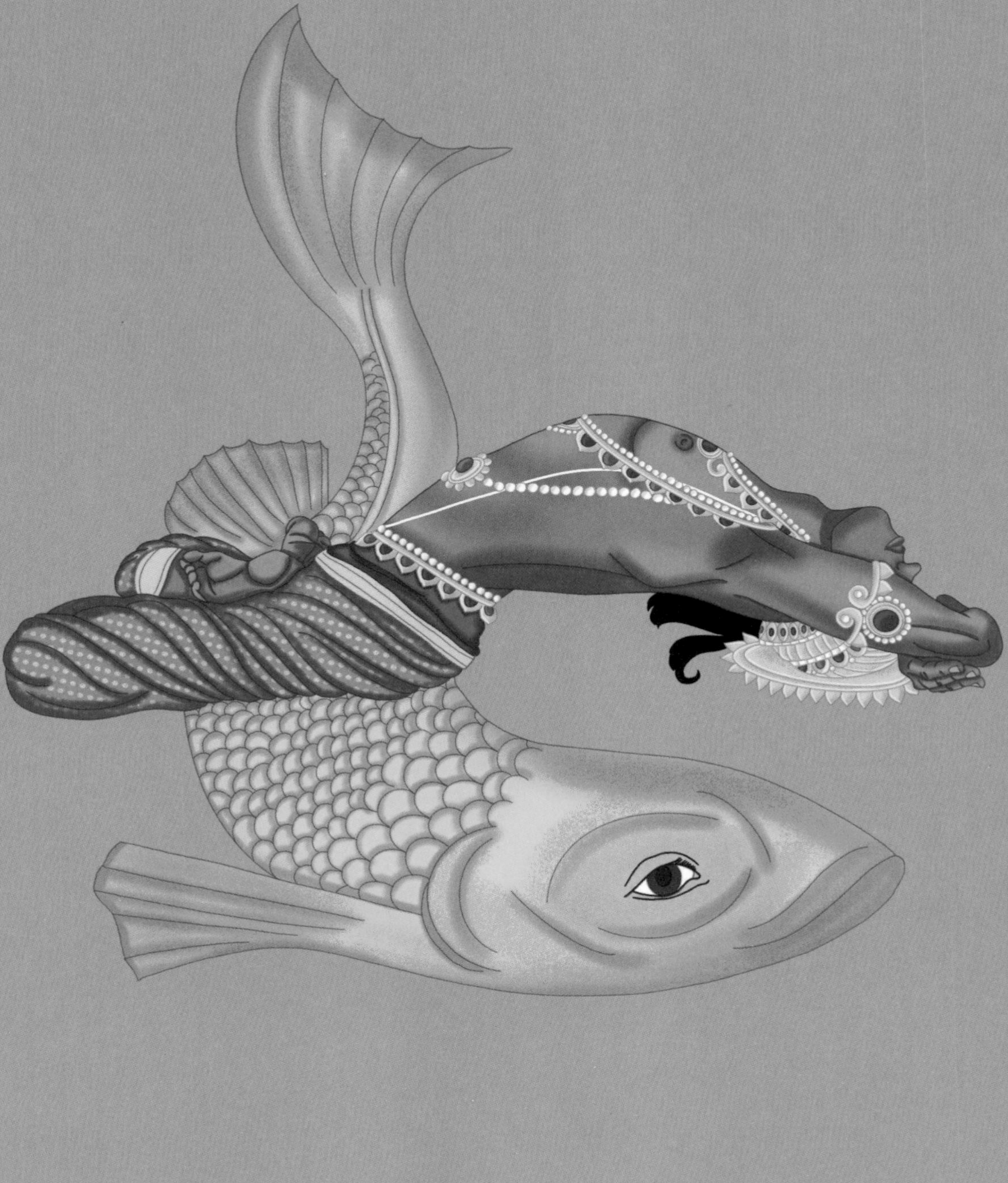

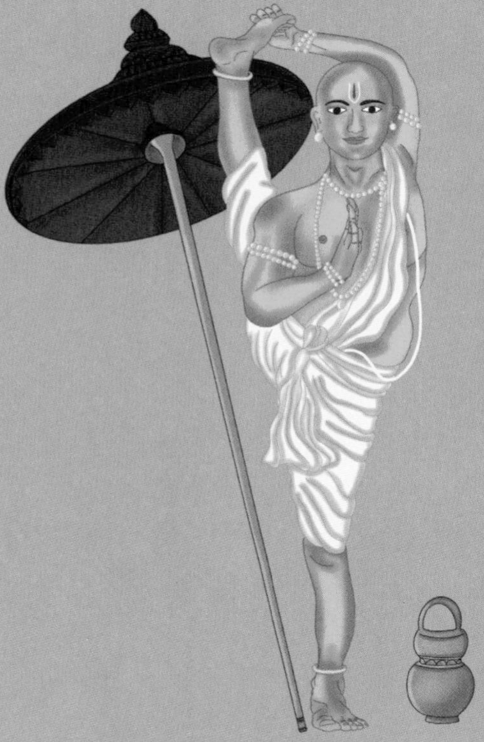

CHAPTER 2

Viṣṇu the Compassionate

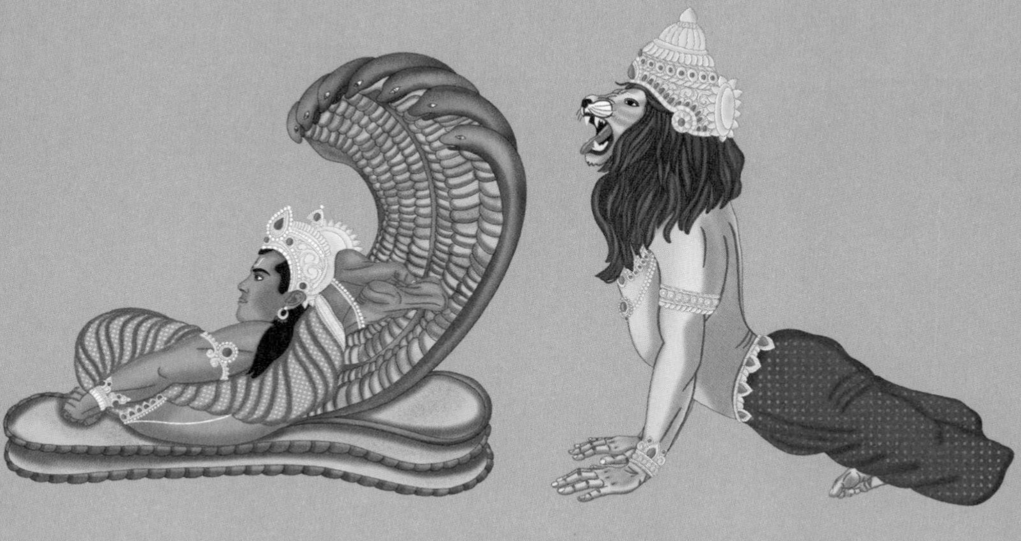

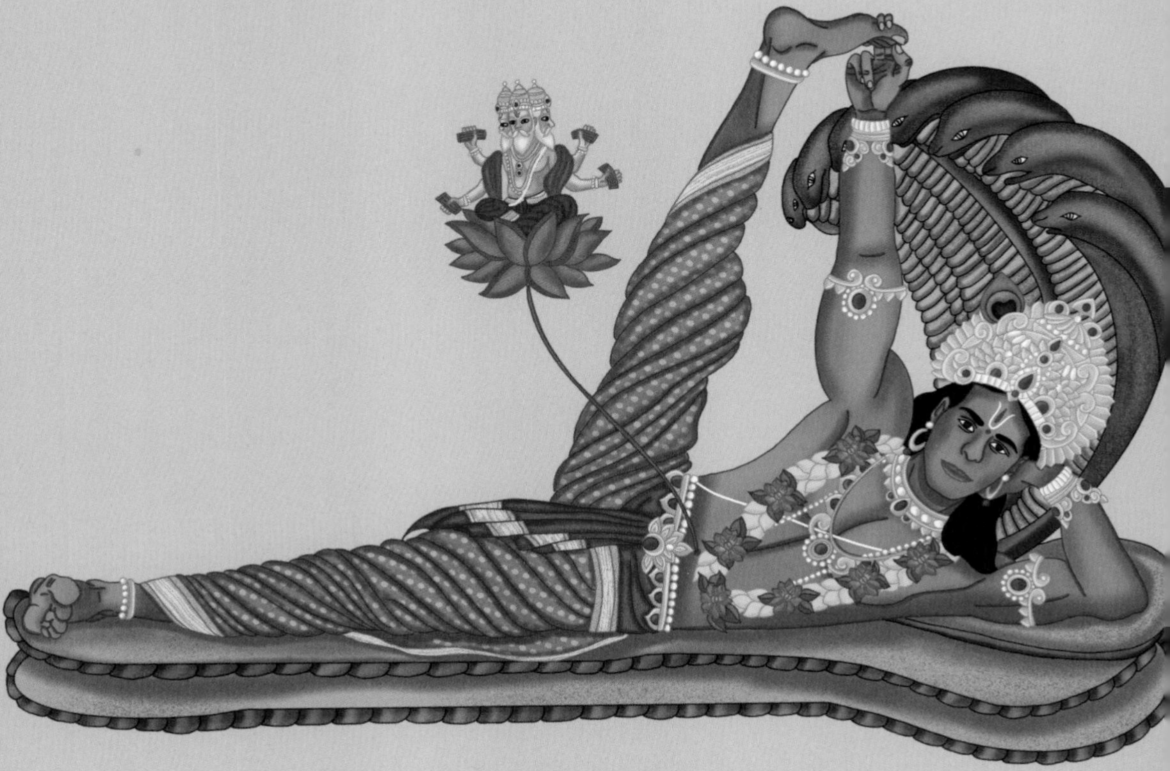

RECLINING POSE
ANANTĀSANA

VIṢṆU'S SERPENT COUCH ON THE COSMIC OCEAN

THEMES
Surrender
Awareness
Balance

IN THE VOID BETWEEN CREATIONS, the great god Viṣṇu sprawls out on his serpent couch upon the primordial oceans. Viṣṇu's cosmic couch is named Ādiśeṣa, the primordial serpent. He, like Viṣṇu, transcends the bonds of time and space, stretched out into infinity upon the oceanic abyss. This abyss is that from which Brahmā creates all things at the dawn of each universe, and that into which Śiva's cosmic dance dissolves all things at the dusk of each creation. The cycles of creation that have occurred before this one, and will occur after it, are without number. It is not that their number is too high to comprehend, rather, they simply lie beyond the very mode of enumeration. They are without beginning (an-ādi) and without end (an-anata). And so, Viṣṇu's great primordial serpent couch is commonly called Ananta—the infinite, he without end. His endlessness can be conceived spatially as well as temporally: Viṣṇu's serpent couch, like Viṣṇu himself, exists beyond the scope of time, space, and causation.

Ananta didn't always have this role. Initially, he was but one of the children of Kadrū, mother of all serpents. His father, Kaśyapa, fathered many species with his 27 wives. Among these were the demons and gods themselves, along with the birds and the snakes. There was a great rivalry between the mother of serpents, Kadrū, and mother of birds,

Vinatā, and there came a time when Kadrū tricked Vinatā into a bet, the loser of which would have to become the slave of the winner. Kadrū won the bet through duplicitous means, with the help of her serpent children. But Ananta would not participate in the vile scheme. He outright refused his mother when she solicited his aid in her nefarious plot. Kadrū was so angry that she cursed him to perish in the fires of King Janamejaya's snake sacrifice. But Ananta was saved by Viṣṇu, and rewarded for his virtue with the honor of becoming Viṣṇu's eternal companion couch.

Serpents and birds are natural enemies, so it is interesting that Viṣṇu adopted both the best of birds, the powerful eagle Garuḍa, as well as the best of serpents, Ananta, as his companions. In describing his own divine supremacy, Viṣṇu's incarnation, Kṛṣṇa, even says, "among serpents, I am Ananta." Garuḍa was Viṣṇu's mount by air, and Ananta his serpent couch when reclining on the cosmic ocean. Garuḍa is a fiery creature; Ananta is watery. Garuḍa is assertive, slicing through air and enemies alike with his talons and sharp beak. Ananta, by contrast, is accepting, supporting the weight of Viṣṇu for all eternity These two special creatures represent two aspects of Viṣṇu: fire and water. Viṣṇu is compassionate, caring, and ready to help. He is the cosmic preserver because he cares so much about creation. He's always available to creatures in need. But Viṣṇu is also virile, powerful, ready to jump into action. His divine discus and mace are always at the ready to battle enemies.

Serpents and Birds have one important thing in common: they are "twice-born," first as eggs, then a second time when they hatch. This is an important nod to Brahminic learning. One is considered twice-born when one is initiated into Vedic training. And so, Garuḍa and Ananta also represent divine knowledge of the mysteries of existence.

Serpents in particular are ancient keepers of esoteric wisdom teachings. The great sage Patañjali, compiler of the Yoga Sūtras, was himself an incarnation of Ananta. Serpent power is associated with kuṇḍalinī śakti, the divine power that pervades all life and the cosmos itself. When localized in the body, kuṇḍalinī travels through the upright spine. Latent kuṇḍalinī power lies coiled in the base of the spine, waiting to be awakened through yogic practice. Patañjali is typically depicted as part serpent, or he is crowned by seven serpent hoods. This represents his raised kuṇḍalinī śakti, piercing his seven chakras, culminating in his thousand-petalled crown chakra. Cobras in particular represent kuṇḍalinī energy, since they are not only serpentine, but can periodically attain upright posture. It is important to note that serpents have no spine, and spend their existences on their bellies. This represents completely latent kuṇḍalinī which has yet to rise. The body is a microcosm of the universe itself, therefore, kuṇḍalinī śakti pervades the cosmos in latent form, symbolized by Viṣṇu's divine serpent couch, Ananta.

Ananta played a very important role when the demons and gods worked together to churn the celestial oceans. The oceans represent existence itself. Viṣṇu took on his great tortoise form and scuttled himself to the bottom of the ocean floor so that the mighty Mount Mandara could be placed upon his back, and used as a churning pole. Just as importantly, Ananta volunteered his own body to be used as a churning rope, and wrapped himself around the great mountain. The gods lined up on one side of the ocean, and the demons on the opposite shore. The demons grasped him on one side and the gods on the other, and their collaborative tug of war began. Great riches were churned from the cosmic ocean, including the Elixir of Immortality itself. And none of this would have been possible without the help of Ananta, representing the kuṇḍalinī power that churns creation in search of immortality.

This posture requires you to be relaxed aware, and deliberate. You need to find your balance, and keep it through relaxed focus. This is how you connect with the power of kuṇḍalini flowing through your spine. But this isn't the active kuṇḍalinī of Garuḍa, this is the passive kuṇḍalinī of Ananta, the primordial serpent support of Viṣṇu. Embody calm, still water instead of fire. Breath into your ruminations upon the infinite, timeless serpent after which this pose is named. There is a space beyond birth, beyond death, beyond the dynamism of time and place. This is the ethereal ocean upon which Ananta expands. This is our innate state. Calm your body, slow your breathing, clear your mind, and surrender yourself, sinking into the power of this posture. Relax the conscious mind and surrender to the depths of instinctive, intuitive knowing.

EAGLE POSE
GARUḌĀSANA

GARUḌA, VIṢṆU'S EAGLE MOUNT

THEMES
Balance
Strength
Centeredness

The great sage Kaśyapa was wedded to 27 of the daughters of Dakṣa, himself the grandson of Brahmā the Creator. Through each of these unions, Kaśyapa fathered a new race of creatures, including the gods and demons themselves. But this is the story of the great eagle, Garuḍa, which begins with two of Kaśyapa's wives in particular, Kadrū and Vinatā. Both were beautiful and loved by Kaśyapa, but quite jealous of each other. Everything was a competition between them. When one attended to Kaśyapa exceptionally well, the other followed suit to compete for his affections. As a matter of fact, due in large part to this competitive spirit between them, they both served Kaśyapa so well that he offered each of them a boon of their choosing. Kadrū asked for a thousand sons of great strength and valor. "So be it!" said Kaśyapa. "You will bear one thousand sons of the serpent race." Naturally, Vinatā had to upstage her rival's boon and asked for two sons whose strength would be greater than that of all Kadrū's sons combined. "So be it!" declared Kaśyapa, "You will bear two stellar sons, both of the race of birds!"

Both Vinatā and Kadrū laid eggs. While Kadrū's thousand serpent sons were soon born, Vinatā's two eggs did not hatch for quite some time. After 500 years had passed, Vinatā broke open one of her eggs. The great bird Aruṇa

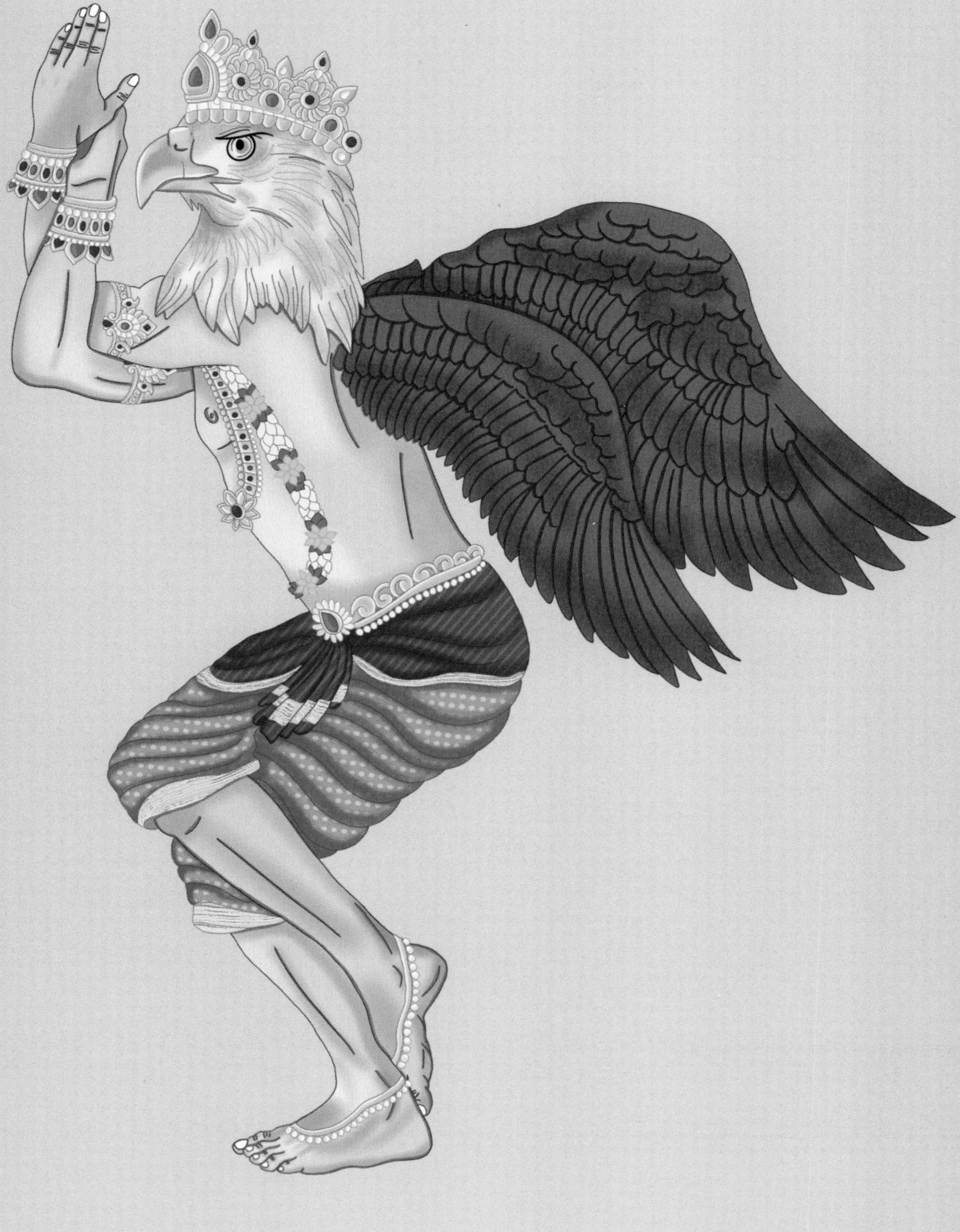

emerged, but so irked was he by his mother's impatience that his first act in life was to lay an awful curse upon her. She would have to wait another 500 years for the other egg to hatch, and all through that time, she would endure dishonorable servitude. Only once her other son was born in proper timing would the curse be lifted. With this, he flew off to serve as the chariot of the sun.

Vinatā's curse came to pass in the form of an ill-advised bet that she was tricked into making with Kadrū. As the loser of this wager, Vinatā was obliged to act as Kadrū's maidservant. But after 500 years of servitude had elapsed, the second egg hatched, and a bird of great magnificence was born. His name was Garuḍa. In accordance with Kaśyapa's boon, Garuḍa was born of the radiance of fire itself; he was ablaze with a luster that rivalled that of the sun. He was the natural king of all birds. Yet, thanks to his mother's gamble, Garuḍa was born into servitude of the snakes and was forced to do their bidding day in and day out. Upon learning of the circumstances under which his mother was tricked into slavery by Kadrū, he approached the serpents to barter for their freedom. The only thing they would accept was some of the Elixir of Immortality, that was kept in the heavens, heavily guarded by the gods. Garuḍa accepted the challenge, and set out for the elixir.

Garuḍa flew up to the heavens and entered Indra's paradise, the abode of the gods, where the elixir was guarded. A great battle ensued, but the gods in all their glory were no match for this fiery son of Kaśyapa. After subduing the entourage of gods, Garuḍa made his way to the sanctuary where the elixir was kept. The sacred substance was surrounded on all sides by pillars of fire. So, he flew to the ocean and, in his great beak, brought back a lake of water with which he quelled the roaring flames. Behind the walls of fire were a deadly contrivance of sharpened and spinning metal blades. But Garuḍa's motion was faster than the wind, and he was able to fly through unscathed. Beyond were two great serpents, who guarded the elixir of life. He beat his great wings, and whipped up a furious dust storm, blinding them, and slew them with his massive claws. Then, he picked up the vessel of shimmering elixir, and took to the skies. Indra, in desperation, launched a fearsome thunderbolt in Garuḍa's direction. But the king of birds was swift and strong, and Indra's weapon was no match for him. He escaped the abode of the gods unscathed, faithfully fetching the elixir to his serpent brothers in exchange for his freedom, and that of his mother.

But as he made his return, a great light came upon him. This was no thunderbolt of Indra, Garuḍa realized—this was more intense, more radiant, and far more powerful. It illuminated the heavens before coalescing before him into the very form of the great god, Viṣṇu the Preserver. Viṣṇu descended to Earth, and Garuḍa humbly followed suit, showing his respect. Impressed by the power and compassion of Kaśyapa's mighty son, Viṣṇu granted Garuḍa a boon. Garuḍa knew that he would soon be free from bondage, and he searched his mind for the right way to use this opportunity. In the presence of mighty Viṣṇu, he realized that a life of service was not necessarily something to be cursed, and asked only that he may be allowed to serve him directly. Viṣṇu was most pleased and decreed that henceforth, Garuḍa would serve as his own *vāhana*: his vehicle.

"And in light of your selflessness," proclaimed Viṣṇu, "I grant you the immortality that your serpent brothers seek." Garuḍa was overjoyed, bowing to Lord Viṣṇu in gratitude. "But now that you are as one of the gods, you must know that one of our prime duties as immortals is guarding immortality from falling into the wrong hands. Much penance is performed in search of the boon of immortality, and no matter what clever loopholes are conceived, immortality can never be conferred to demons, men, or snakes."

Seeing through the lens of an immortal, Garuḍa understood the importance of guarding the elixir from less worthy beings. He saw that they would otherwise have all eternity to wreak havoc upon heaven and earth. He understood that in order to gain the upper hand with his serpent half–brothers, he would have to trick them. So, as promised, he delivered the nectar to the serpents, and gained freedom for himself and his mother. But as he handed it over, he suggested the serpents may wish to ritually bathe, to purify themselves before imbibing the elixir. Fancying themselves pious, they took the bait, and as they bathed, Viṣṇu took the elixir back to the heavens and again fortified it. He knew that Garuḍa alone had the strength and skill to break through the gods' defenses, but he now possessed the wisdom to never do so again.

Garuḍāsana calls you to reverently clasp your hands in anjali mudra. *You are also called to withdraw and coil together arms and legs to connect with your core strength. In order to maintain this posture, one needs to be fully centered, focused, balanced. Imagine yourself riding a powerful eagle across the heavens, finding stillness in the flight.*

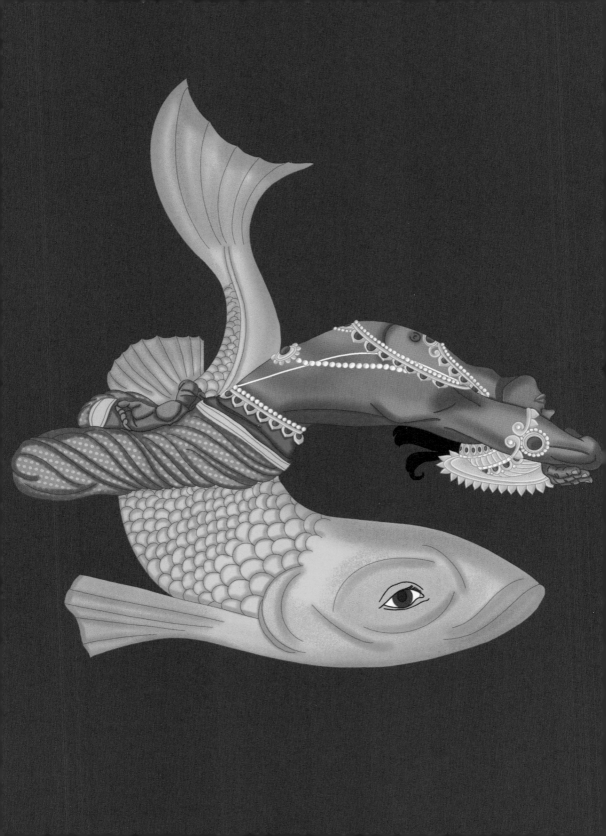

FISH POSE
MATSYĀSANA

VIṢṆU'S FISH INCARNATION

THEMES
Relaxation
Reverence
Stability

LONG AGO, MANU, THE PRIMORDIAL MAN, was carrying out his sacred ablutions in the holy Ganges River, when along came a tiny fish. The fish politely asked Manu to protect him, lest he be eaten by the bigger fish. Manu agreed to protect the little fish, and carried him home within a fistful of water, cupped in his hands. Having arrived, he placed the fish in a little jar and tended to him. As time passed, the fish grew, and needed a bigger jar, and eventually, a tank. In due course, the fish became too big even for the tank, and so, Manu carried him back to the Ganges. The fish thanked Manu for protecting him and nurturing him, promising to repay the favor one day. Manu was gratified that the fish had grown large and strong under his care, and visited it in the Ganges every day when going to perform his sacred rituals. To Manu's astonishment, the fish kept on growing with each passing day until he was so large, he could scarcely swim in the Ganges, and needed to swim to the ocean.

"Great fish," Manu addressed him, "certainly you are no ordinary creature. Who are you, and why have you come into my care?"

"Manu, you are correct—I am no ordinary creature," stated the fish. "I am Matsya, Viṣṇu himself, incarnated as a fish to fullfill my divine purpose here on Earth."

Manu bowed before the banks of the river, honored to be in the presence of the lord. "Hail Viṣṇu, Lord of the Universe!" he proclaimed. "I am honoured that you have selected me to nurture you to maturity in this incarnation of yours. But please tell me Lord Matsya, why have you incarnated into this world in the form of a fish?"

"For everything there is a purpose, Manu. Every creature has its own skill. It is only as a fish that I may fullfill my divine duty to protect humankind. No other creature but a great fish can accomplish the task before me. And you have well passed your test. As a reward for your kind protection, you will be protected a thousandfold."

"Lord, what danger befalls me, and how will you protect me?" asked Manu, simultaneously reassured and alarmed.

"There is a great flood coming to drown the earth, Manu. The beasts of the earth will perish in this great deluge. Only in my fish incarnation can I save creation. Go forth, Manu, and build a great ark in which you will secure the finest seeds and animals of the earth. Bring yourself, your family, the Seven Seers and the divine Vedic revelations. With these you will rebuild and populate the world once the waters subside. I will meet you at the mouth of the Ganges when the rains commence." With that, Matsya swam away. Manu prostrated on the banks of the Ganges in wonder and awe at what had just transpired.

Manu went back and commenced construction of the great ark as Matsya instructed. It was of massive dimensions, strongly built, and well insulated against the elements. The ark was filled with the finest seeds and animals of all creation—birds of the air, and beasts of the land. Manu also gathered the Seven Seers and told them of the impending danger. He honored them well and beseeched them to join him, which they did. The Vedic revelations had been etched upon their hearts, memorized and internalized, so as not to be lost during the great deluge.

No sooner had the Seven Seers entered the ark than the rains began to fall. At first, they were mild, then moderate. Then the rains grew heavy and hard. Lightning and thunder filled the heavens as torrents of rain pelted down upon them. They were all grateful to be in the ark. As the thunderstorms began in earnest, great Matsya appeared before them. He had grown still larger, and was now twice the size of Manu's ark. He instructed Manu to tie a rope around his horn and attach it to the ark, which Manu did. The waters continued to rain down destruction, swallowing the earth and all its creatures.

Matsya pulled the ark, navigating the turbulent waters with grace and ease as the storm raged on. He pulled the great vessel to the top of the Himālayas , which appeared as a tiny island surrounded by the rising waters. They weathered the storm there until it passed. All breathed a sigh of relief as the waters began to subside, and the earth reappeared before them. Matsya advised the entourage that the storm had passed and they could emerge. Looking out upon them, Viṣṇu assumed his divine form and addressed them thus:

"For protecting a tiny fish, you've been protected from this great deluge, Manu, first of men. Go forth and repopulate the earth, for it has been saved by my grace. I have fullfilled my duty to protect creation through my divine fish pose. I will return again, as dwarf, lion, and man to protect the world when it is imperilled. I bless you to repopulate the earth, and build a society founded on the divine Vedic revelations. And most importantly, Manu, never forget to protect the imperilled as you protected me when I was a tiny fish. The imperilled, like me, are divine in flesh, and worthy of protection."

All hailed the great god Viṣṇu until he vanished. They then set out to do as he said, and repopulate the earth.

When doing this pose, remember the dharma of Viṣṇu: support of the world. Relax into the posture knowing you are supported by the forces of the universe, and attain a state of stability as an embodiment of Viṣṇu's Matsya avatāra *incarnation who preserved creation through the great deluge.*

TORTOISE POSE
KŪRMĀSANA

THE CHURNING OF THE COSMIC OCEAN (PART I)

THEMES
Withdrawal
Stillness
Support

EONS AGO, THE UNIVERSE WAS SO NEW that many of its elements had yet to come into existence. Creation was so young at this point that immortality itself had yet to grace the cosmic stage. It was a time when the Devas (divinely lustrous beings) were at perpetual odds with their discordant, divisive counterparts, the Daityas. Although these two classes of being were of one primordial lineage—both having been fathered, though through different mothers, by the great sage Kaśyapa, grandson of the Creator himself—they continually opposed each other, vying for control over the cosmos. Since even the heavenly beings were mortal in this ancient age, there was great anxiety among them, for, should one group win a decisive victory, it would result in annihilation of the other forevermore.

In the interest of securing the welfare of the Devas, Indra, king of heaven, sought counsel from the Creator, Grandfather Brahmā himself. Since Brahmā was the ultimate progenitor of all of creation, he must have insight on how to proceed with the predicament at hand. Indra travelled to Brahmā's realm and prostrated himself before him in humble respect. He told Lord Brahmā of his woes, and Brahmā consoled him, assuring him that there was hope.

"Abandon all anxieties about death, O King of Heaven. You can overcome mortality through immortality. I have

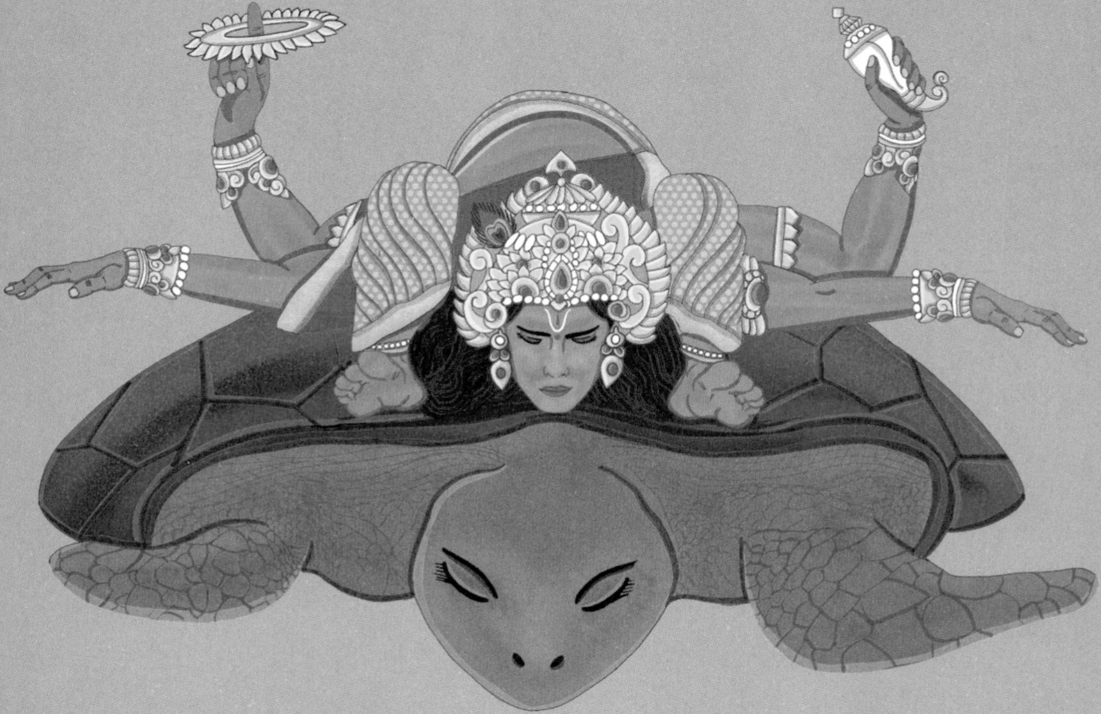

provided for all things in this grand creation, so immortality itself can belong to you and the rest of the Devas, Lord Indra! I have created hundreds of billions of universes, and each and every one I blessed with everlasting life, for those who seek it."

"Wonderful, wonderful, Great Grandsire!" exclaimed Indra, relieved. "Tell me where to find immortality and I shall retrieve it without delay!"

At this, Brahmā let out a knowing chuckle, "Retrieve it? How can you retrieve what has yet to exist?"

"But I don't understand, Grandfather. You said you had created it! Have you not?"

"I merely said I had provided for it. It is you who must manifest it by your own efforts. I have imbued the fabric of the cosmos with the seeds of all experience, but these seeds mostly remain in potential. All beings must reap and sow. You must fulfil your duties in the grand scheme of things, and only then shall you receive what is coming to you. These are the laws of dharma and karma by which the role of all beings in this universe of mine is determined."

"Forgive my haste, Lord Brahmā," said Indra, "but how then shall I churn the Elixir of Immortality for the welfare of the gods?"

"You must churn the entire cosmic ocean—the whole Milky Way! There is no other option."

"But that would be a colossal task, surely more than one mere Deva such as me, or any one being, could possibly undertake. I would have to amass all the gods for this monumental feat!"

"Indeed," agreed Brahmā, "and do not forget, in your self-centeredness, Lord Indra, that you Devas represent only half of my progeny—only half of my strength. You Devas alone would only be able to churn half the ocean. And, like churning only half a pot of milk, how would the butter emerge? To churn all of creation would require the collective strength of Devas and Daityas alike. This is the only way to immortality. You gods must embrace your shadows, and work with them." And with those wise words, the great god vanished, leaving Indra behind, dumbfounded.

Acting on the advice of Lord Brahmā, the Devas devised a plan to engage the Daityas to work with them to procure the Elixir of Immortality. But, in secret, they planned to cheat the Daityas out of their share and keep the elixir for themselves. Indra knew that this dark deceit would be the only way to safeguard his throne, and the welfare of the beings of light.

Indra informed the Devas of his plan, and succeeded in eliciting the aid of the Daityas, whose desire for immortality was just as strong. All beings quickly gathered. The Devas assembled and lined themselves up on one side of the Cosmic Ocean, and the Daityas assembled on the other side of its enormous banks. Vāsuki, king of the serpents, volunteered his very body as a churning rope, wrapping himself around Mount Mandara, which was to be used as their churning pole. But though they had their rope and pole, the gods had nothing steady to place the pole upon, that the great mountain may be turned, and the cosmic ocean, churned. Seeing what must be done, Viṣṇu manifested himself as a tortoise and plunged himself down to the ocean floor. He withdrew inside his shell, into utter stillness, and offered his back for the mountain to be placed upon. The gods rejoiced in gratitude, and the churning began.

Compassionate Viṣṇu is the Preserver deity, in charge of preserving the universe at all costs. By incarnating as a tortoise, Viṣṇu took the form that was needed, as he always does. The tortoise represents a state of focused sense-withdrawal, as its head and limbs are drawn into its shell. It has a silent, grounded inwardness. Viṣṇu's tortoise teaches us that this highly advanced state can be of great service to those around us. By withdrawing awareness from the senses, one can offer strong, sturdy support and, much like Viṣṇu's tortoise avatāra, *can become the support of the world itself. In this myth, it is upon the back of the steady and stationary tortoise that treasures are churned form the cosmic ocean. Likewise, it is through the practice of this state of withdrawal that the treasures of life can be accessed, for you and those that you support.*

This story is continued on page 39.

LION POSE
SIṂHĀSANA

NARASIṂHA, VIṢṆU'S LION INCARNATION

THEMES
Poise
Confidence
Assertion

THE GODS ARE ALWAYS TRYING to bring about unification throughout creation, while the demons seek always to divide it. But though the gods prize purity of spirit, they are not without their trickery, and though the demons are always up to something, they are not without their virtues. Throughout the ages, many demons have performed monumental acts of penance, in order to achieve their ends. There was one such demon, an arrogant and bitter being named Hiraṇyakaśipu—a sworn enemy of the great god, Viṣṇu the Preserver. Viṣṇu had killed Hiraṇyakaśipu's brother, and to make matters worse, his own son, Prahlāda, had then become a devotee of Viṣṇu, and prayed to him every day, without fail. In his vengefulness, Hiraṇyakaśipu set out to elevate himself to godlike status. Like all demons, he longed for immortality, believing that if only he could live forever, his son would worship him, and not his fated enemy.

So, Hiraṇyakaśipu devoted himself to the worship of Śiva. For centuries, he went without food and water and, with steadfast devotion, chanted Śiva's sacred syllables and meditated on his divine form. Eventually, Śiva was pleased by Hiraṇyakaśipu's zealous penance, and appeared before him.

"Hail Mahādeva, great God! Glory to the blue-throated Destroyer of the universe!"

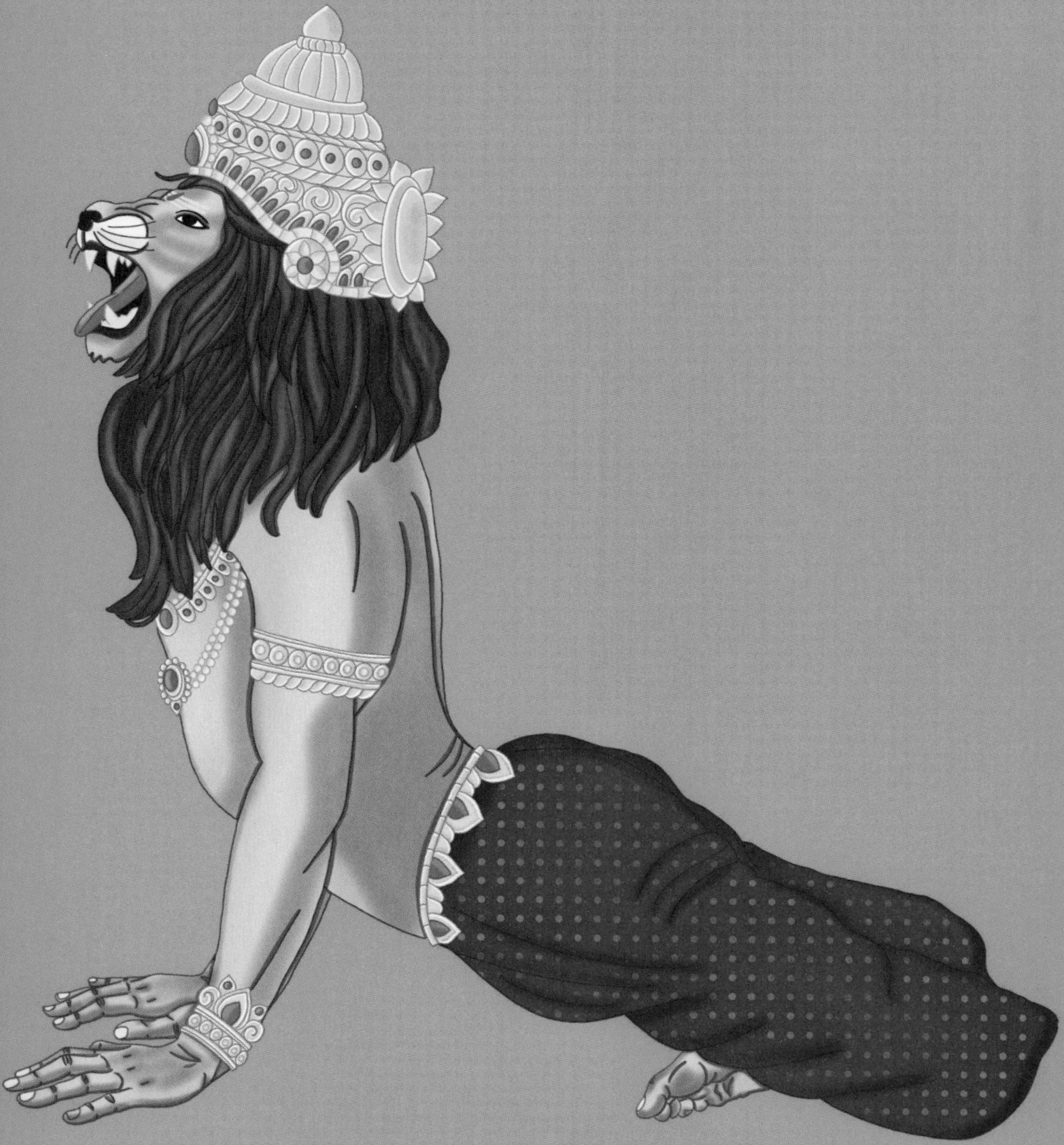

Śiva replied, "You have duly earned a boon, great demon, for your steadfast penance. Name it and you shall have it! Though of course, be mindful that the same stipulation applies for all who seek a boon: you cannot wish for immortality."

"Great Śiva, that was precisely the boon I sought! For as you know, the gods have cheated us out of our share of the elixir of life! Had they not done so, my brother would still be alive."

But Śiva was unmoved, replying, "I will grant anything you wish, except for immortality."

Reflecting for a moment, the demon's face lit up as an idea came to him. Pleased with himself, Hiraṇyakaśipu gave voice to his clever wish: "May I be slain neither at night, nor by day, not by man, god, nor beast, neither indoors nor outdoors, neither on the ground nor in the air! This is my boon, great God." With a twinkle in his eye, Śiva granted the demon's wish, and then disappeared. The demon was giddy with satisfaction and excitement. Surely, he had tricked the mighty Śiva into granting him immortality. He returned to his abode, swollen with dizzying pride.

Upon his return, Hiraṇyakaśipu heard the familiar sound of his son's melodious voice chanting the holy names of Viṣṇu at the home shrine for his dusk prayers. Drunk with his newfound power and outraged at his son's insolence, he burst upon the shrine and interrupted Prahlāda's prayers.

"How dare you worship that pathetic excuse for a god?" he shouted. "Do you fawn over him because he is an immortal? Well today your father, too, is immortal! I've just been granted a boon by Śiva!"

But Prahlāda was calm, responding, "Father, demons cannot attain immortality. It goes against the grain of creation. Surely you know this."

"Insolent fool! I have asked the Lord Śiva that I may not be killed by day nor night, neither indoors nor outdoors, not by man, beast, or god, neither on earth nor in heaven! What more does one need to attain immortality? Viṣṇu is no longer greater than I, so you will stop worshipping him at once, and worship me instead!"

"Viṣṇu is not merely immortal, father," Prahlāda quietly persisted, "he pervades the universe, existing in every crevice of creation. I will worship him for the rest of my days, father, and you should do the same."

"Are you truly so foolish, child?" asked Hiraṇyakaśipu, his voice trembling with anger, "Viṣṇu is everywhere, is he? Well, I suppose he's in this pillar over here too then, is he?" He radiated a thick air of contempt. But Prahlāda remained unperturbed.

"Lord Viṣṇu is in the pillar. He is here and everywhere, father."

Mad with rage, Hiraṇyakaśipu grabbed Prahlāda by the hair and dragged him to the pillar, shouting, "Well, let's crack your head against the pillar and see if Viṣṇu comes out!"

It was in that very moment, as the faithful Prahlāda's skull was about to be smashed against the pillar, that the stone itself cracked open, and a blinding burst of blazing light shone forth from it. The blaze coalesced into a ferocious form—half man, half lion. It was Viṣṇu in his Narasiṃha form, incarnate, not fully god, man or beast, but somewhere between the three. He gripped Hiraṇyakaśipu and dragged him forcibly into the threshold—neither inside, nor out—where it was precisely sunset—neither day, nor night. He lifted him off the ground, and slaughtered him in midair with his powerful claws. As the sun set, so too came the ending of Hiraṇyakaśipu's short-lived immortality.

Hiraṇyakaśipu's story is one of misplaced energy. He spent centuries trying to outdo and overcome Viṣṇu, rather than allow himself to be protected under the cover of his power to preserve. The gentleness of Prahlāda granted him access to the fierce loyalty and unhesitating protection of Viṣṇu's most punishing incarnation. When enacting this pose, connect with the self assurance and grace of the leonine energy for which it is named. Be bold and unafraid to summon the lion's ferocity in accordance with your dharma.

THREE-STRIDES POSE

TRI-VIKRAMĀSANA

VĀMANA, VIṢṆU'S DWARF INCARNATION

THEMES
Strength
Stance
Expansion

ONCE, THERE WAS A GREAT DEMON named Bali who had succeeded in conquering all of the underworld. Satisfied with himself, he sent his forces into the light of day and conquered kingdom after kingdom until he held dominion over the whole wide world. Proud and powerful, he coveted even more territory. So, Bali launched a campaign against the throne of heaven itself. He combatted Indra, Lord of Heaven, and his forces long and hard until, at last, he reigned victorious, lord of the three worlds. Never before had a demon conquered so much of creation.

Bali was quite pleased with himself. So much so, he started offering people boons to display his power and superiority over them. Drunk with power and fancying himself a god, he would offer property, riches, food, finery, whatever people wanted! After all, he now possessed all of the wealth in the three worlds.

Indra and the gods, cast out of heaven, visited the abode of the Creator, Lord Brahmā, for guidance.

"Grandfather," began Indra, awakening the Creator from his cosmic trance. "Bali has conquered the three worlds and we gods are again cast out of heaven! How could this be?"

"Everything happens for a reason, Lord Indra. For every problem there is a solution, and every solution brings with it blessings upon creation."

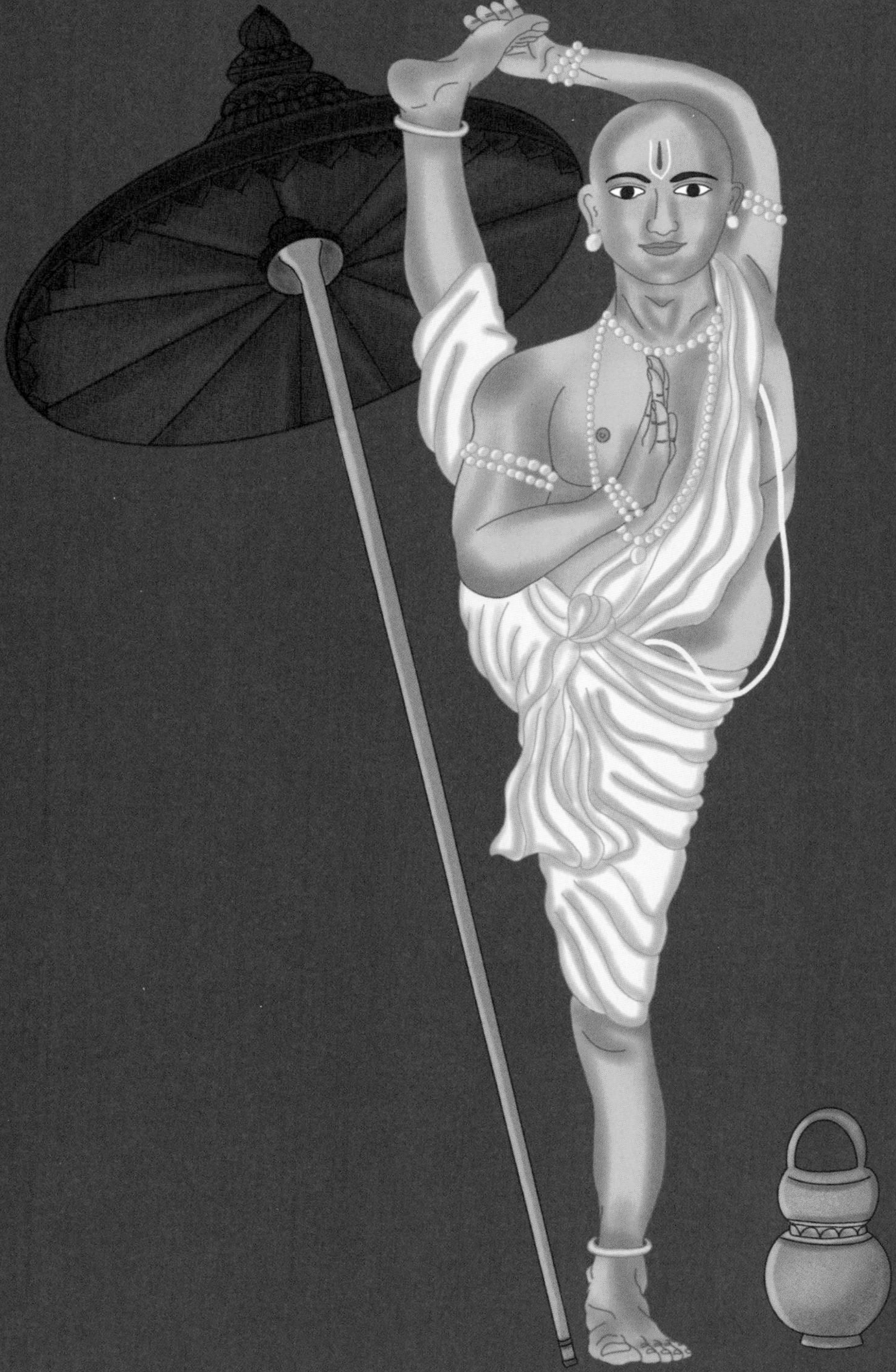

“That’s all good and well for philosophical types, Grandfather, but how do we get our power back? Surely, as Creator, you must know.”

“When I wake from my meditation to speak with you, I am, like you, a mere cog in this creation of mine. All of us individuated beings have but a limited perspective. And so, I possess only part of the puzzle. We are more than mere puppets to the whims of destiny—we co-create the universe through our actions. I do not know how to solve your problem, but I am sure that Śiva will know.” With that, Grandfather Brahmā returned to his cosmic trance and the gods departed.

The gods visited the abode of Śiva, Lord of Yoga. He too was in a cosmic-trance state which, though similar to Brahmā’s in practice, was oriented toward a quite different purpose. Brahmā’s function is to create, and so when he’s done, he retires to divine meditation for the duration of creation, only interrupted here and there to confer a boon or offer advice to those who’ve come for such. But Śiva’s function is to destroy the cosmos at the end of time, and so he spends much of his time in divine trance, accruing the power that he will need in order to do so. His yogic meditation is likewise interrupted every now and then to confer a boon, find a solution, or to spend time with his beloved consort Śakti. While Indra and the gods were fine with waking Brahmā from his trance, they dared not wake Śiva, for fear of incurring his colossal wrath. So, they waited patiently in the presence of the meditating lord.

Luckily, Indra and the gods did not need to wait long. Lord Śiva was in a merciful mood. He sensed their presence, and opened his celestial eyes, bringing his awareness to the scene at hand.

“Glory to Śiva! Hail to the Blue-Throated Lord!” exclaimed the gods, in reverence.

“Welcome, gods of heaven, to my mountainous abode. I know of the situation in the three worlds, and what brings you here. It is true what Grandfather Brahmā has told you—we all have a role to play, yet this role is not mine. I do know, however, that Viṣṇu will be able to help you. It is his dharma to preserve creation against evil, even if he needs to incarnate personally as man or beast on earth. Travel to his abode and you’ll find your solution.” The gods thanked Lord Śiva, paying their respects before setting out for the abode of Viṣṇu, the last of the three great gods.

Lord Viṣṇu warmly received Indra and his entourage, hearing their concerns. He then assured them that he would devise a plan and bring resolution to the situation. Viṣṇu incarnated in his dwarf form, Vāmana, and paid a visit to the court of the demon Bali, planning to appeal to his vanity.

"O great conqueror of the three worlds, it has been told to me that you are offering boons to we lowly citizens of Earth. May I request three strides worth of land from you?"

"Ha! Of course you can, dwarf! What is three puny strides of land to the king of heaven and earth? So be it. Pick your three strides and they shall be yours."

But then, Vāmana extended his stature, growing as big as a full-size man, then a giant, then a tree. He kept growing and expanding until he was the size of a mountain, then as tall as the sky itself. With one stride, he covered all of the earth and the underworld, and with his second stride he claimed the heavens.

"Bali, I've made only two strides, and now there's nowhere left for me to step! What do you suggest I do in order for you to fullfill your gracious boon?"

In wonder and awe at the figure now towering over creation, he knew it must be none other than Lord Viṣṇu himself, come to teach him humility. He was indeed humbled, and abandoned his hubris.

"Hail, Lord Viṣṇu! I realize my arrogance in thinking that the conquest of land could compete with your divine sovereignty. The power I wield over the three worlds cannot compete with the divine power you wield, Lord! I offer my head for you to take your third stride."

And so, with this, Viṣṇu smiled at the wisdom of Bali, and placed his foot on the demon's head, liberating him from the cycle of rebirth. The balance of power was restored throughout the three worlds, and Viṣṇu was praised in his dwarf incarnation as Tri-Vikrama, he who took three steps.

When pride and hubris are allowed to take charge, be it within or without, great ignorance and foolishness abounds. When dealing with such inflated arrogance, call upon the humble form of the dwarf. Remember how it is to be small, before you tap into the expansiveness that is also yours to embody. Dignity and humility are the difference between grandeur and grandiosity. When you engage Tri-Vikrama pose, call to mind the grandeur of Viṣṇu, resisting the pull of overconfidence, and remembering the eventual humility of Bali.

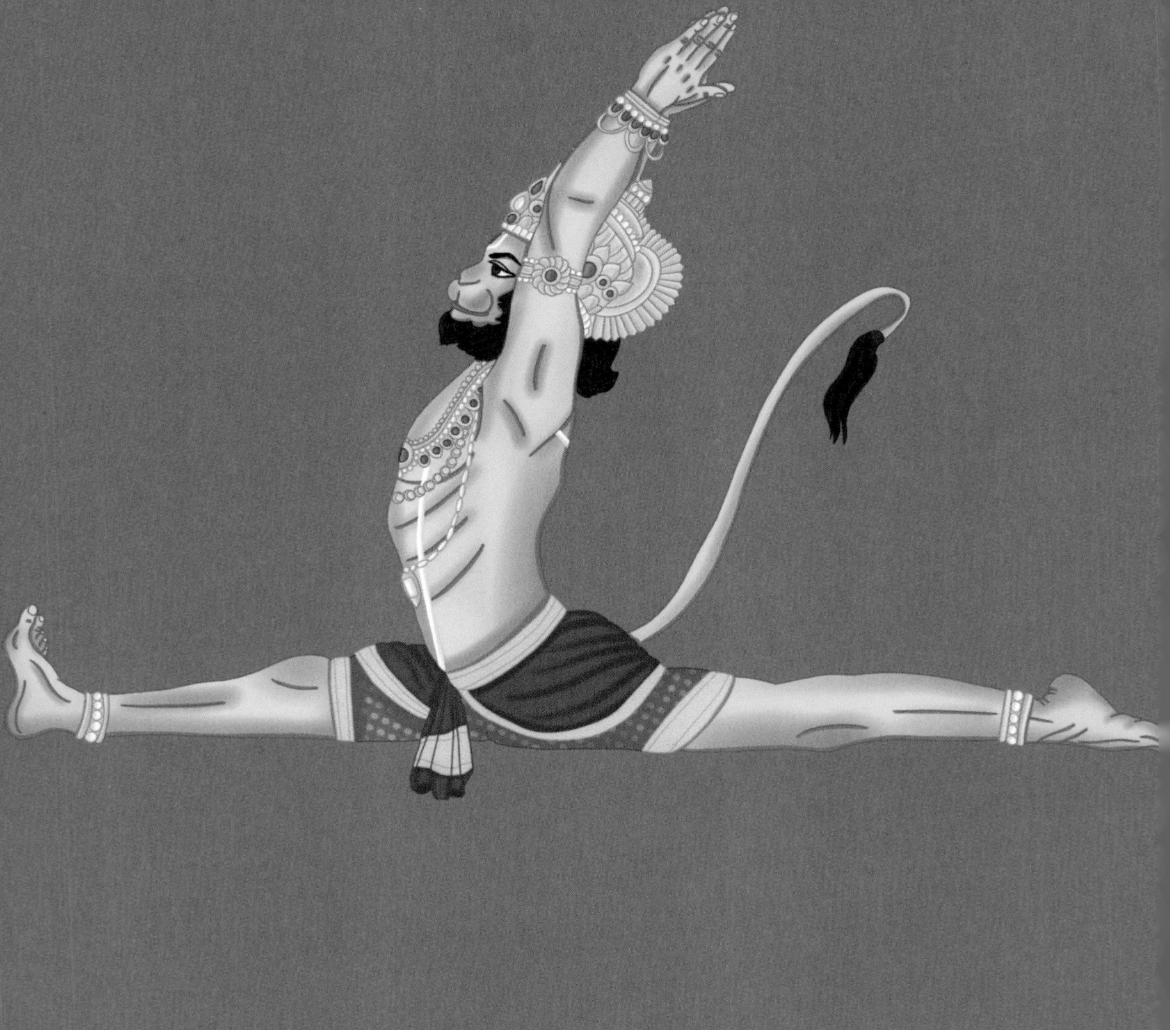

MONKEY POSE
HANUMĀNĀSANA

THE LEAP
OF FAITH

THEMES
Reverence
Faith
Possibility

There was once a great prince named Rāma, who was an incarnation of Lord Viṣṇu. At one time, Rāma was made to undertake exile in the forest for 14 long years. Accompanying him in the forest was his wife Sītā, and his faithful brother Lakṣamaṇa. They all renounced royal life to live as forest hermits for the duration of their exile.

While there, Rāma discovered a sophisticated race of simian beings living in great cities in the middle of the forest. These monkey-people called themselves the Vānaras. Greatest among them was Hanumān, unmatched in strength, speed, and loyalty; he was no ordinary monkey-man. Hanumān was son of the wind god Vāyu, hence his great strength and speed. He was the first of the Vānaras that Rāma met while roaming the forest, and there was an instant spark between them. Theirs was a powerful soul connection, so much so that the instant they met, Hanumān knew in his heart that he was meant to serve and protect Rāma for the rest of his days. Hanumān pledged his allegiance and loyalty to Rāma, who gladly accepted it, since the love between them was mutual.

Once, while in the forest, the demon-king Rāvaṇa kidnapped Rāma's wife, Sītā, and carried her off in his flying chariot to live in captivity on his faraway island kingdom of Laṅkā. Sītā greatly despaired at the separation from Rāma.

Rāma too was in shock and despair and was inconsolable for some time. Then, pulling himself together, with Hanumān's help, he launched a search party to find Sītā. The Vānaras were at Rāma's side every step of the way. They divided themselves up into three groups: one to venture north, one east and one west. The greatest area, to the south, Hanumān offered to cover alone, seeing as no entourage would be able to match his speed, and would only slow him down.

Weeks turned into months, and the three search parties came back empty-handed. Meanwhile, Hanumān had reached the southern tip of India, also without any sign of Sītā. He gazed with dismay at the seemingly unending sea before him. Hanumān knew of the island kingdom of Laṅkā and he knew he must venture there to look for Sītā before returning empty handed. But he had no means of crossing the sea. If only he had a boat! He doubted he would ever be able to cross the ocean and complete his task. And yet he had pledged allegiance to his beloved Rāma, so he must find a way! The powerful Hanumān sat on the banks of the sea and kneeled in prayer, asking for divine inspiration for the impossible task ahead of him.

Hanumān was not only physically strong, but also possessed tremendous strength of character. Faith and devotion are true tests of strength. He prayed to his father, the wind god, and asked for help, gently cupping his hands, that he might receive whatever grace may descend from the heavens. Then he knew what he must do. He gathered his strength, and summoned every iota of faith he could muster, chanting the name of Rāma all the while. Then he backed up, and took a running leap toward the horizon. He kicked off with his back foot as his front foot pierced the air in from of him. In a split posture, defying gravity, he hurled himself through the air, propelled by the power of belief, and fueled by grace. The great leaping monkey succeeded in crossing the sea, flying above the waves, and landing on the soil of Laṅkā. He took a moment to offer his thanks to the divine for helping him realize the true extent of his abilities, and carried on to find Sītā in the court garden. She was delighted to hear news of Rāma's search, and he was delighted to have fullfilled his duty to bring news back to Rāma of his beloved Sītā. Thanks to Hanumān's faith, loyalty, and bravery, Rāma was able to learn of Sītā's whereabouts, marshall a great army, and fight a long and arduous war to win back her freedom.

We are more than we think we are, and with effort and faith, we can realize this potential. Hanumān is a powerful symbol of this realization. Like all of us, he is a primate through and through. And yet, through his faith and devotion, he is able to sublimate his animal impulse to attain divine status. Hanumān is peaceful, only exerting force in times of need to protect the imperilled. Also, Hanumān is a lifelong celibate. Through the sublimation of his libidinal forces, he's able to attain considerable spiritual power, which affords him great wisdom and strength. Whenever you see Hanumān in iconography, notice that his tail is raised. A tail, like a spine, stems from the root. Hanumān's raised tail is a symbol of his raised kuṇḍalinī power. We, too, can sublimate our base impulses and raise our awareness from the beastly to the divine. We too can transmute our animal instinct into great love, devotion, and spiritual power. When you engage this posture, remember the steadfast devotion of Hanumām which garnered the grace to render the impossible, possible.

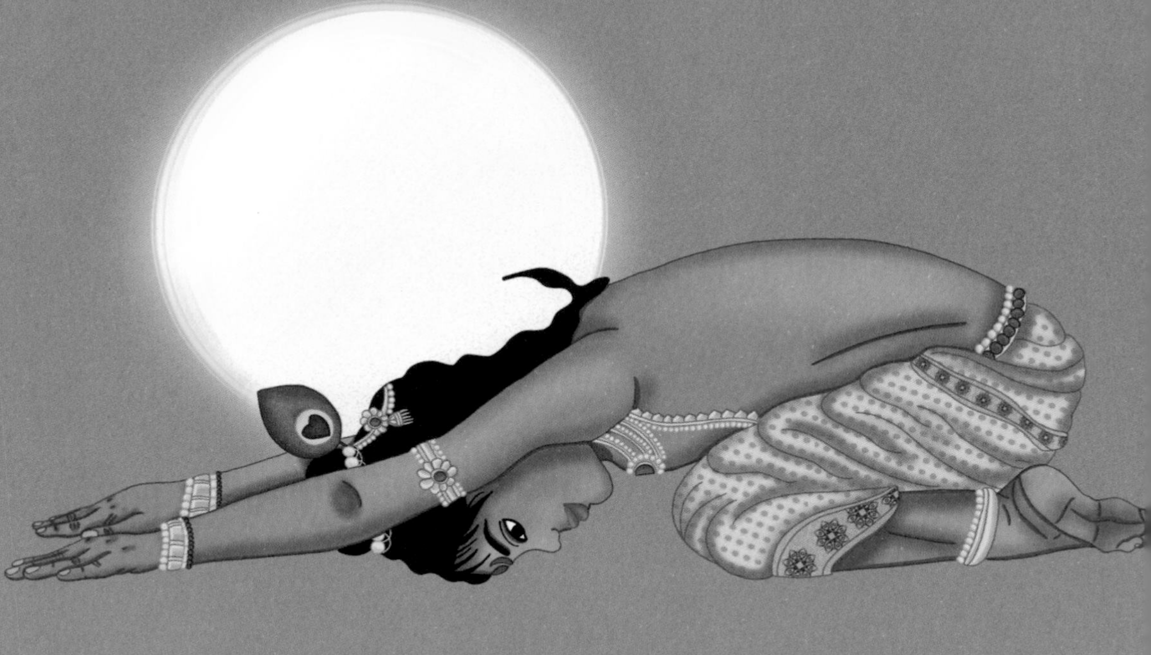

CHILD POSE
BĀLĀSANA

KṚṢṆA'S
DIVINE PLAY

THEMES
Grounding
Safety
Serenity

One day, when Kṛṣṇa was still a little boy, he and his older brother, Bālarāma, were playing in the yard with some of their friends. Bālarāma noticed that Kṛṣṇa was eating dirt and ran inside to tattle on him and fetch their mother, Yaśoda. Yaśoda ran out in haste and prepared to intervene.

"Have you been eating dirt?" Yaśoda asked Kṛṣṇa. Kṛṣṇa vigorously shook his head. "Are you sure about that?" Yaśoda pressed on.

"No, I haven't," muttered Kṛṣṇa, with dirt covering his lips and cheeks.

"Kṛṣṇa, we've talked about your naughty pranks," scolded Yaśoda. "Now, are you very sure you have not been eating mud?" Kṛṣṇa vigorously shook his head once more.

"Alright," said Yaśoda with as much sternness as she could muster in the face of her adorable son whose face was covered in dirt, "open your mouth then!"

"Are you sure you want me to do that?" he asked.

"Yes, I'm sure. Enough stalling. Now open up!"

Kṛṣṇa grinned, then opened his mouth to let Yaśoda look inside. She indeed saw dirt in his mouth and was about to reprimand her adorably mischievous child, when she was stopped in her tracks. The tiny mound of dirt grew to the size of her entire yard, then a field, then an entire hillside.

Yaśoda saw within Kṛṣṇa's mouth the great continents and oceans of Earth, and then the scene grew even grander. She saw the sun, the moon, and planets. She then beheld the dizzying array of stars and galaxies whirling about in the universe. She was utterly mesmerized, witnessing the rise and fall of the cycles of time in her son's mouth, and the lives of all beings past, present, and future. She even saw herself looking into her son's mouth! Inebriated by this cosmic vision, she realized her son was no ordinary being. He must be none other than Lord Viṣṇu, Preserver of the universe himself, having taken on incarnation in the body of her precious son. Kṛṣṇa must be part of some divine play for the restoration of righteousness on Earth.

Finding herself enveloped in Kṛṣṇa's mouth, she saw the lord himself manifest before her, radiant, beaming.

"Hail Viṣṇu, Lord of the Universe!" exclaimed Yaśoda. She then bowed reverently before the divine form of Viṣṇu. "How may I serve you, Lord?"

"You are already serving me, mother Yaśoda," declared the lord. "For having incarnated as Kṛṣṇa, yet a child, I need the divine love and protection only a mother can give. There is no greater dharma in the universe than protecting those who need it. And for this, I bless you a thousandfold for your maternal sacrifices and care."

"Lord, I will have to be more respectful to my son, knowing he is your incarnation. Please forgive my disrespect in scolding Kṛṣṇa."

"Yaśoda, you'll do nothing of the sort!" Viṣṇu replied, "Kṛṣṇa is as human as he is divine, and needs the loving discipline only a mother can give. The roles you play are all part of the divine play, for a higher purpose. And so, I will grant you a boon at this time. I will bless you to forget what you have learned today, since in forgetting, you'll be able to attain your greatest joy in this life: being Kṛṣṇa's mother." Yaśoda thanked the Lord for his compassionate gift, praising the play of the gods.

She then found herself back in the mundane world, in her yard looking into her child's mouth. She swiftly removed the dirt that was in there, scolding him for his naughty tricks. Kṛṣṇa simply grinned. Surely Kṛṣṇa must have been hungry, reasoned Yaśoda, which is why he was eating dirt. So, she picked him up, gave him a kiss on the forehead and took him inside for a snack. Kṛṣṇa was delighted, as was Yaśoda.

The parity between Viṣṇu's divine and child forms is also found in the story of the great sage, Mārkaṇḍeya, whose meditation was interrupted by a torrential downpour. The end of the world was near, and the cosmic deluge had begun. The earth was soon covered in water. Atop a massive wave, Mārkaṇḍeya spotted a mystical banyan tree, somehow thriving despite the flood. Upon approaching it, he saw a babe in one of the banyan's branches. Mesmerized, he approached the child only to be swallowed by his inbreath. Much like Yaśoda, Mārkaṇḍeya witnessed the cosmic expanse unfurling within the mouth of the child. Mārkaṇḍeya realized it must be none other than Viṣṇu entering his yogic slumber at the end of the age. Like Yaśoda, he was returned from the mouth of the child. The difference between the stories of Mārkaṇḍeya and Yaśoda is that Mārkaṇḍeya did not forget the experience. As a sage, he was conscious of the revelation before him and remembered it. Yaśoda forgot what she was shown by divine ordinance, so that she could carry out her role in the divine play.

One important concept in the world of Indian philosophy is that of līlā (play). This doctrine views mundane reality as resulting from the play of the divine. In this narrative vignette, one sees the divine play specifically superimposed on child's play. Play is not a mundane thing. It occurs when children feel safe and lose themselves in the moment. We have much to learn from children in this respect. In many ways, the spiritual question is one of regaining our childlike mindset within the context of a more matured awareness. When engaging this pose, connect with the calm grounding of a child who feels safe and content. Appreciate both the innocence of the child, able to play when they want, and the diligence of the mother who keeps them so safe.

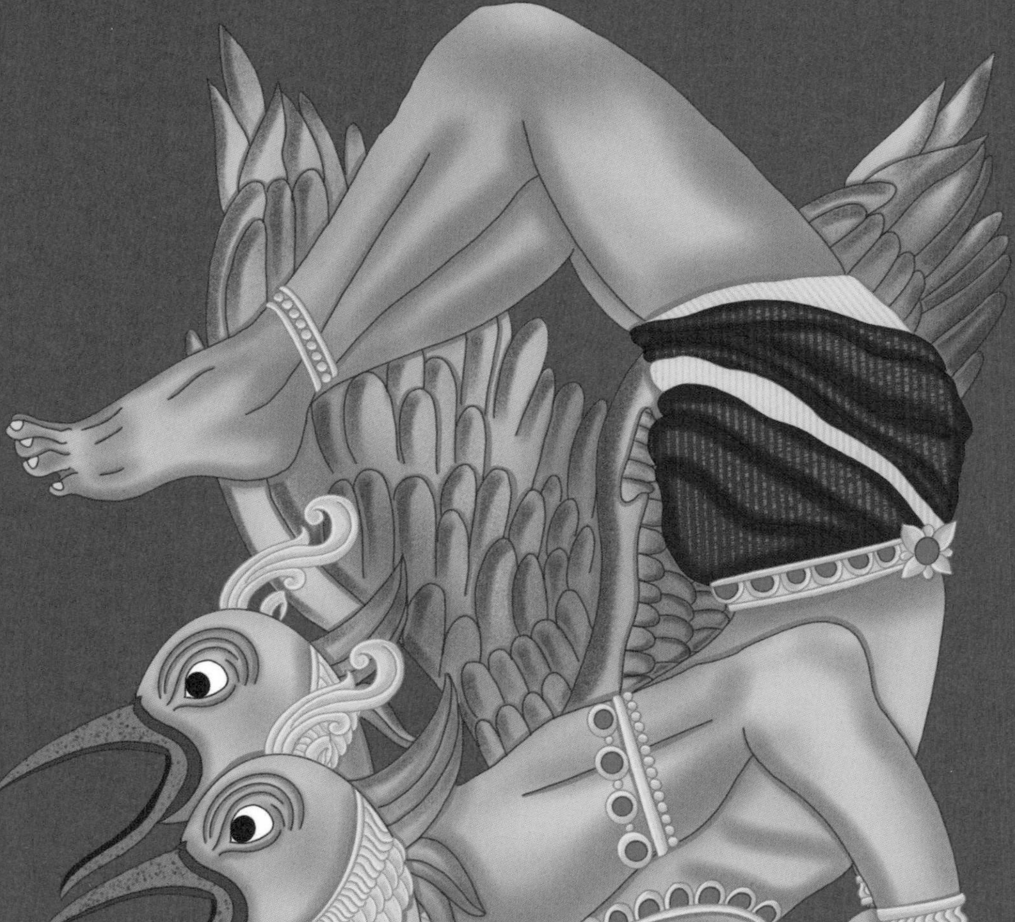

TWO-HEADED BIRD POSE

GAṆḌA-BHERUṆḌĀSANA

THE TWO-HEADED EAGLE

THEMES
Challenge
Reciprocity
Wrath

Once, the demon Hiraṇyakaśipu performed great penance from Brahmā and earned a boon. He wanted was immortality, but immortality is reserved for the gods, and no demons may attain it. Like most demons in his position, he attempted to ask for a clever boon that would, in effect, grant him immortality. So, he wished to be killed neither by day nor by night, neither indoors nor outdoors, neither by god, man, nor beast. Brahmā granted the boon, knowing all too well that such boons will only hold up for so long. In order for this demon to be killed, Lord Viṣṇu had to incarnate as Narasiṃha, half-man, half-lion. Since he was neither fully man, lion, or god (but a combination of all three), he would qualify to slay Hiraṇyakaśipu. But what about the other conditions? Viṣṇu, (Narasiṃha) dragged Hiraṇyakaśipu to the threshold so he was neither indoors nor outdoors, and ripped him apart at twilight, neither during the day nor at night. And that was the end of the demon Hiraṇyakaśipu and his hubris-fuelled boon.

However, as Narasiṃha ripped apart Hiraṇyakaśipu, the demon's blood entered his lion's mouth and, having tasted it, Narasiṃha developed an insatiable bloodlust. Viṣṇu forgot his divinity and hunted far and wide to indulge his taste for blood. Seeing the gruesome state of affairs, the gods paid a visit to Brahmā the Creator, and asked for his aid.

"Grandfather Brahmā, you must do something! Viṣṇu the Preserver has forgotten who he is and prances about the earth devouring prey!"

"Yes, I have seen with my divine eye what has happened upon the destruction of Hiraṇyakaśipu. Usually, I send you to see Viṣṇu when there's an issue to be sorted out. He is, after all, the Preserver! But who preserves creation when the Preserver is out of commission?"

"Then all is lost!" cried the gods.

"There's always a way, my children. All one needs is some creativity to find it. And luckily, being the Creator, I have plenty of that to go around!" The gods were calmed by this and, becoming curious, they asked:

"But if the Preserver is imperilled, who then can we call upon to do the preserving?"

"There are many paths up the mountain, so to speak," replied Lord Brahmā, with a twinkle in his eye. "One man's destruction is another's preservation. Destroying a destructive force amounts to preservation, doesn't it? So, go see the great Destroyer, Lord Śiva, who will be able to put an end to Narasiṃha's carnage."

With that, the gods all travelled to Śiva's abode and informed him of their woes. Seeing how dire the situation was, Śiva transformed himself into a terrifying creature, assuming his Śarabha form: a leonine creature with two heads, two wings, eight legs and a long serpent's tail. Śarabha descended to Earth to engage in a gory battle with Narasiṃha. The two fought fiercely before Śarabha dealt the crippling blow to Narasiṃha, going straight for his jugular. Thus, the Narasiṃha incarnation was destroyed and Viṣṇu was freed. He immediately realized his divinity and returned to his celestial duties, praising the greatness of Śiva.

However, having tasted the blood of Narasiṃha, it was Śarabha who now suffered from intense bloodlust. Śiva forgot his divinity and wreaked havoc upon the earth. Given the ensuing chaos, the gods again returned to Brahmā.

"Grandfather Brahmā, you must do something!" complained the gods again. "Śiva the Destroyer has now forgotten who he is and prances about the earth devouring prey!" exclaimed the gods.

"Well," replied Lord Brahmā, "just as one man's destruction is another's preservation, so too is one man's preservation another's destruction!"

"Grandfather, please stop speaking in riddles and tell us what to do!"

"Must I explain everything to you gods?" sighed Brahmā. "Well, just as the Destroyer Śiva was called upon to destroy Narasiṃha for the sake of preservation, so too should you call upon the Preserver Viṣṇu to preserve the earth by destroying Śarabha!"

"But wasn't it Viṣṇu's incarnation as Narasiṃha that got us into this situation?" asked the exasperated gods.

"Yes, but it is Viṣṇu's dharma to incarnate on Earth as man, beast, or whatever is required to protect the earth, and I'm sure he will do so, having learned from his past experience." So, the gods went off to find Viṣṇu and tell him about the problem at hand.

Upon hearing how dire the situation was, and feeling responsible, Viṣṇu was determined to help. He knew he must incarnate in a form powerful enough to compete with Śiva's Śarabha incarnation. So, Viṣṇu assumed his terrifying Gaṇḍa Bheruṇḍa form, the great two-headed bird with colossal power, capable of skewering an elephant with a single talon. Gaṇḍa Bheruṇḍa descended to Earth, to the place where Śarabha was wreaking havoc. A cataclysmic battle ensued between the two celestial beasts, after which Gaṇḍa Bheruṇḍa reigned victorious, clawing Śarabha to death. This time he made certain to use only his talons, safeguarding his beak from imbibing any of Śarabha's blood, thereby breaking the cycle. Viṣṇu's conquest over Śarabha released Śiva from this dreadful form, causing him to remember his divine nature. Śiva returned to his abode, praising Viṣṇu, just as Viṣṇu had praised him before. Viṣṇu also returned to his own abode, glad to have returned the favor, and to have fullfilled his divine purpose to preserve the world.

As you do this difficult pose, remember the difficult task of Gaṇḍa Bheruṇḍa, who had to conquer the fearsome Śarabha—an incarnation of Śiva that was created to conquer his own previous rampant incarnation, Narasiṃha. Remember too, the cyclical nature of the story as you attain a circular posture, with your feet reaching your head in the most unexpected and challenging manner. It is also crucial here to remember the interplay between preservation and destruction as well as the collaboration of Śiva and Viṣṇu. They each have a past. So, before you answer the question whether Viṣṇu is supreme, or Śiva is supreme, remember the tale of this two-headed bird, who may view the answer differently from each pair of eyes.

YOGIC SLEEP POSE
YOGA-NIDRĀSANA

VIṢṆU'S SLUMBER

THEMES
Inwardness
Awareness
Energy

VIṢṆU REPRESENTS COSMIC CONSCIOUSNESS. He is the awareness that pervades creation. Hence, he is creation's Preserver. But when Śiva performs his divine dance of destruction and the universe is dissolved back into the primordial ocean, Viṣṇu sprawls out into infinity upon his celestial serpent couch Ananta, and falls into a deep, meditative sleep—his *yoga nidra*. This state is beyond the waking state, and beyond the dreaming state as well. This is a deep and dreamless sleep where the mind is silent. This is where Viṣṇu retires once the cycle of creation has been completed. He reawakens when, by the grace of Lord Brahmā, a new cycle dawns. Creations rise and fall like waves on the cosmic ocean, without beginning, without end. As time and space themselves are dissolved into that primordial ocean, there is no "place" for Viṣṇu to retire to, only a "state" of consciousness—his yogic slumber. Almost all souls remain in a state of suspended animation until the dawning of the next creation, for only one embodied being has ever been able to survive the cosmic dissolution: this is the story of the great sage, Mārkaṇḍeya.

Mārkaṇḍeya's parents were childless and so they performed great penance to Śiva in order to obtain a son. Śiva granted their boon, but told them they could either have a wise, noble son who would live 16 years, or a deceitful and

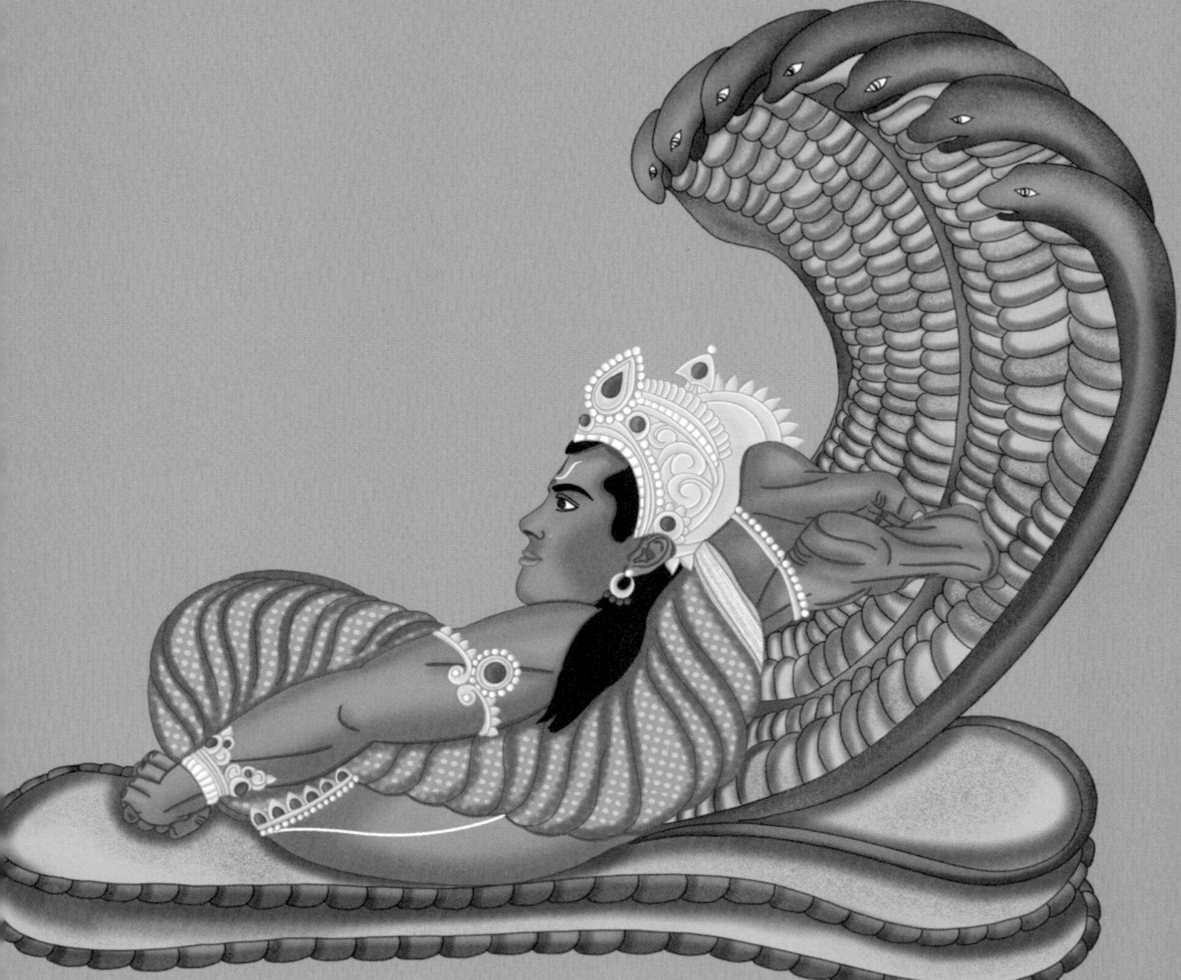

insignificant offspring who would live to the age of 100. The couple chose the first option, and the great sage Mārkaṇḍeya was born. Toward his 16th birthday, his parents began to weep. They confessed the circumstances of his birth, but the wise Mārkaṇḍeya was unphased.

Fully accepting that all creatures must die, Mārkaṇḍeya set out to worship Śiva for the remaining time he had left on Earth. He performed rituals, chanting the sacred mantras before the holy Lingam stones at one of Śiva's many temples. When the appointed hour had arrived, Yama, the god of death, came to ensnare Mārkaṇḍeya in his infamous noose. But as he gathered in his rope, he saw that he had captured not only the young sage, but also the Lingam stones that he had been worshipping at. Śiva appeared and dismissed Yama, granting Mārkaṇḍeya the boon to eternally remain 16 years old. Mārkaṇḍeya was grateful to Śiva, and went on to be a great world teacher.

After millennia of teaching and blessing people on Earth, Mārkaṇḍeya retired to deep meditation for the remainder of the age, becoming oblivious to all that was around him. Then, one day, he noticed a strong gust of wind, which grew in intensity. Torrential rain began to fall. The storm became a hurricane. The rivers soon overstepped their bounds and inundated the land. Whirlpools formed and a great flood was upon the earth. Mārkaṇḍeya was tossed and turned by the tempestuous waves about him. From the crest of a very tall wave, he spotted a great banyan tree, glowing magnificently, and untouched by the storm. He was drawn by the dazzling splendor of its mysterious presence, and fought his way toward it in reverence and awe.

As Mārkaṇḍeya approached the banyan, he noticed that its radiance was coming from one single branch, though it was enough to illuminate the entire tree. Looking even closer, he saw that it was, in fact, an infant, nestled amid the branches, which so lit up the scene. Mārkaṇḍeya drew closer, mesmerized by the glowing child. The child laughed playfully, and with one of his inhalations, Mārkaṇḍeya was sucked into his mouth. The sage was awestruck to behold the sun, moon, stars, and great galaxies within this infant's mouth! He saw too the landscapes of earth—mountains, forests, deserts, tundra! Every known flora and fauna and class of creatures populated the infant's mouth!

The ages went by in the twinkling of an eye. Mārkaṇḍeya was left breathless by this divine vision. Then, as swiftly as the child's breath had sucked him in, his exhalation pushed him back out, and he found himself, again, in the presence of the great banyan tree.

Mārkaṇḍeya beheld the child again, and knew he must be in the presence of the great god Viṣṇu the Preserver. The storm that had raged around him was, he realized, the destruction of all things, the dissolution of space and time, and the ending of the age. In the abyss between universes, in the time between ages, Viṣṇu gathers the essence of all creation into himself for their protection, knowing that nothing can survive such ultimate and complete destruction. But Śiva's boon had rendered Mārkaṇḍeya immune even to his own destructive forces unleashed in fullness. So Mārkaṇḍeya knew then, he had been called toward the great god Viṣṇu so that he himself may be preserved.

This posture is emblematic of the divine child from Mārkaṇḍeya's vision, coupled with Viṣṇu on his serpent couch in yogic slumber. This is a pose that calls one to withdraw one's awareness, to become more compact, to go within. The "sleep" you are called to is not a state of unconsciousness, but a state of altered consciousness. You are to fall asleep to the mundane world, and your attachments therein. Viṣṇu slumbers upon his serpent couch, Ananta, which represents dormant kuṇḍalinī, sleeping until it is activated at the dawn of creation. Similarly, advanced yogīs will feel kuṇḍalinī energy flowing through their spine in this pose. But this energy is not to be expended at this time. Rather, it is to be acknowledged, relished, and internalized, for it will be needed at the dawn of your own creation.

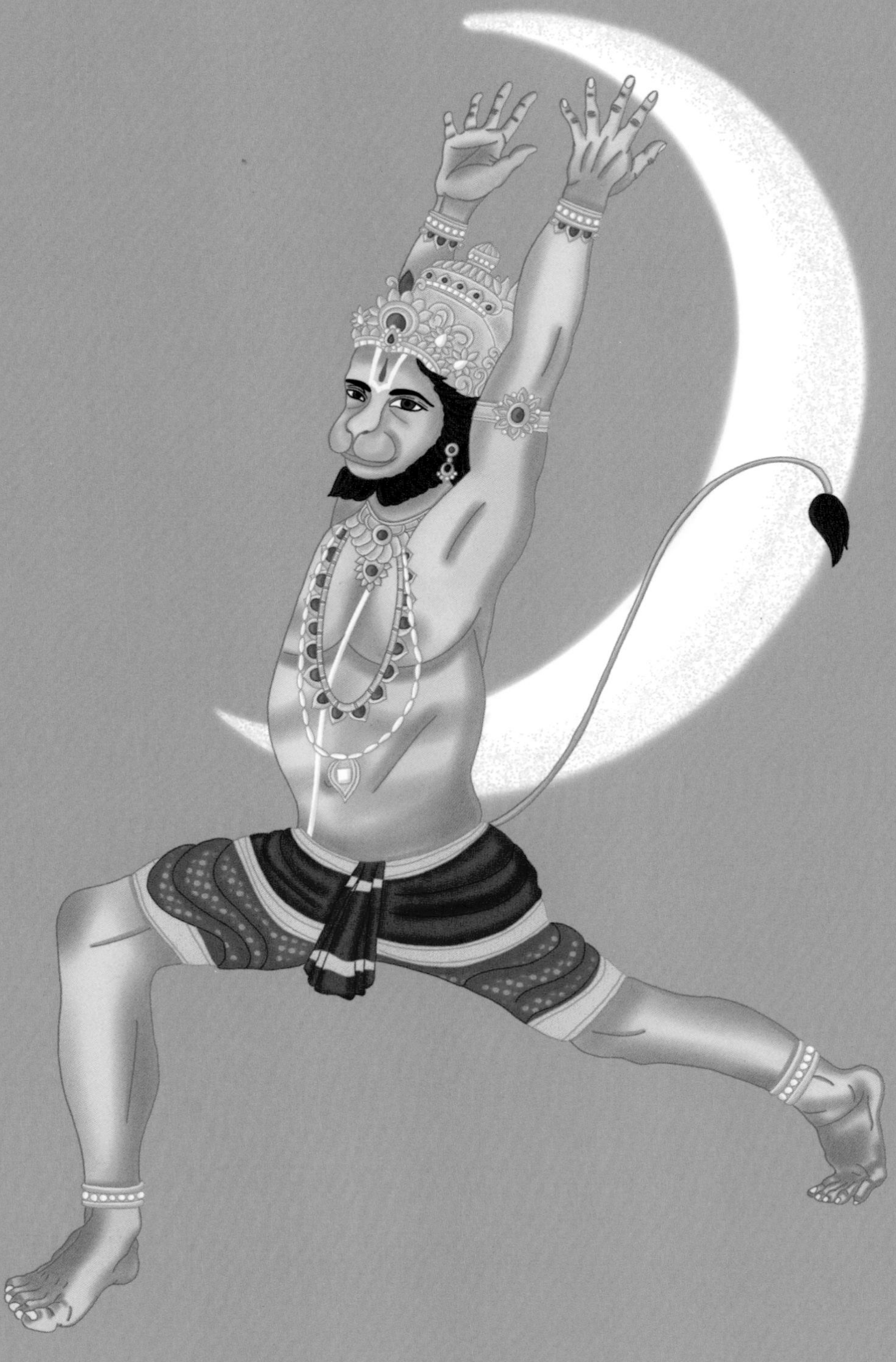

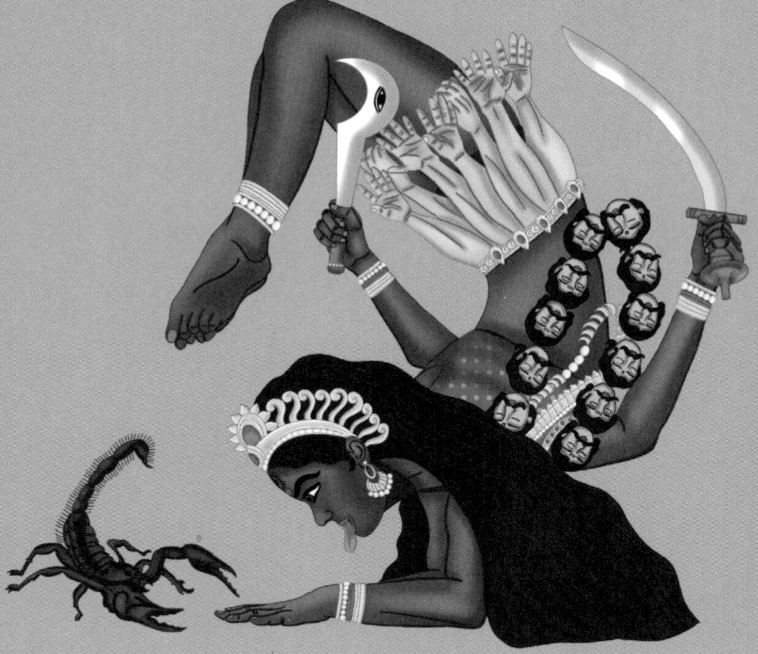

CHAPTER 3

Devi and Her Manifestations

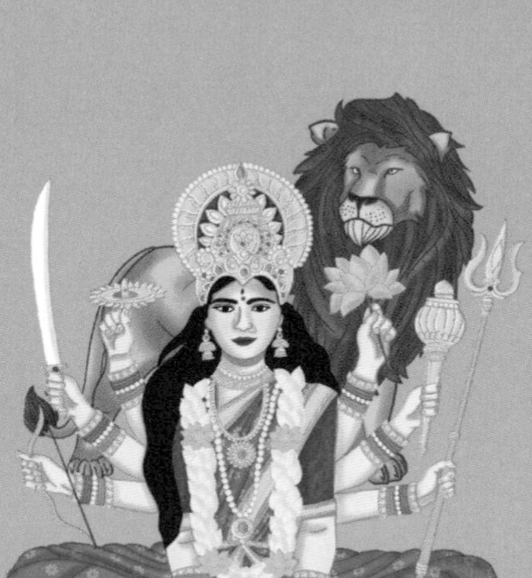

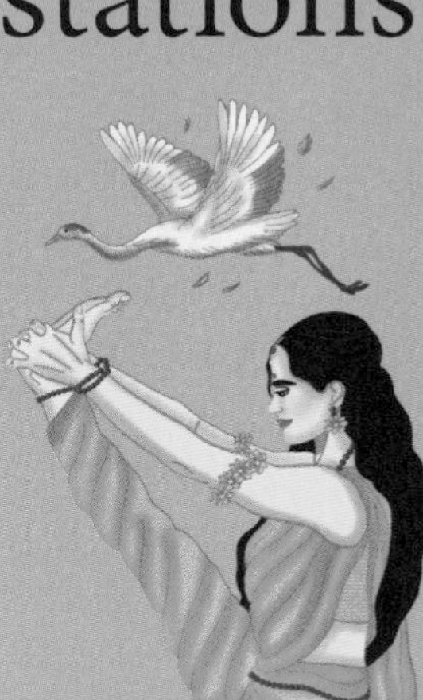

SWAN POSE
HAṂSĀSANA

SARASVATĪ,
SACRED SOUND

THEMES
Lightness
Clarity
Striving

AT THE BEGINNING OF TIME, the Creator god Brahmā looked out onto the primordial oceans, surveying the scene. At the end of the previous cycle of creation, all things had been dissolved into the ocean by Śiva's blissful dance of destruction, and now it was up to Brahmā to initiate a new cycle. By the power of his will, time and space unfurled before him. But he could not get anything else to manifest. The scaffolding of the universe was erected, but he was at a loss as to how to proceed.

Brahmā took a moment to himself, turned inward, took a deep breath and expanded his consciousness to receive what he could from the cosmic abyss. Every god has a role to play in the cosmic dance, but the scope of the cosmic consciousness that governs all things is mysterious, even to the gods. As Brahmā meditated, inspiration struck! He opened his mouth, took in another deep breath, and let out a cosmic "oṃ" sound. The sacred sound pervaded the very corners of the universe. At the end of his utterance, to his utter astonishment, a majestic, four-armed, feminine form was born of his mouth. She was glistening, majestic, milky white and shining like a thousand suns.

"Great goddess!" Exclaimed Brahmā. "Who are you and how did you manifest before me? I haven't even created anything yet! All I've done is utter OṂ!"

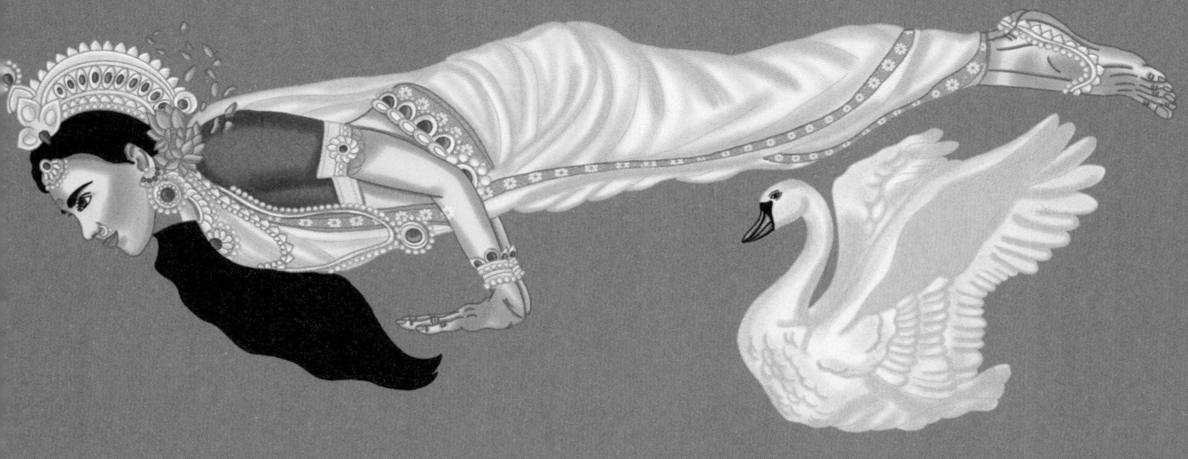

"Lord Brahmā, I am Sarasvatī, divine inspiration. You prayed for inspiration, and you have received it. I exist beyond space and time, uncreated and undestroyed by the cycles of creation, preservation and destruction. I am the divine, cosmic white noise of the universe. I manifested before you by virtue of your divine utterance, of which I am an embodiment. I am the sacred sound with which you will create all things."

Brahmā was delighted to be so inspired by Sarasvatī, and glad to be able to proceed with the unfurling of the universe. The two embraced like peas in a cosmic pod. Brahmā and Sarasvatī—Creator and Creativity—communed as one to create the cosmos. Inspired by Sarasvatī, Brahmā uttered mantra after sacred mantra to create the galaxies, stars, and planets. Even more subtle mantras were spoken to create the laws that govern creation. Their divine dance resulted in the birth of everything within the universe. When creation was in order, the communion of Brahmā and Sarasvatī culminated in the creation of the Seven Seers, noble and wise, to be entrusted with all divine knowledge for the welfare of the world.

Sarasvatī schooled the seers about the primacy and power of sound: "Sound is the most subtle, and most sacred of the five elements, Seers. Most dense is earth, of which is born your sense of smell, less dense is water, the medium of taste. More subtle is fire, which ignites sight, and subtler still is air, which propels touch. But sound is most subtle of all, dwelling in the ether element. Don't mistake the sound you hear through air as the totality of sound. You Seers will have to use your subtle senses to hear ethereal transmission."

The seers were in awe as Sarasvatī taught them how to tune into subtle vibrations. She guided and inspired them to channel the sacred sounds innate to the cosmos. Day in and day out, they received sacred revelations, which they coded in Sanskrit, the language of the gods. "You must memorize the sounds you hear," schooled Sarasvatī, "for in memory alone will these sacred sounds be embodied and live through you. From memory can a verse be uttered aloud, indeed intoned. Writing will not do for the divine word. It is the residue of the embodied experience. The text is on the tongue! Inscribe these sacred cosmic sounds within your hearts and minds. Let them purify and nourish you, as they will for all whom incant them." The seers learned well from Sarasvatī and codified and preserved her wisdom in the form of the Vedic revelation. They set up teacher-student lineages through which this learning, the grace of Sarasvatī, flows to this day.

Sarasvatī is inspiration itself, required for deep learning and artistry alike. She is summoned by poets to serve as their muse, and by all engaged in study. She is the patron goddess of knowledge, wisdom, and the arts. Because of her connection with the sacredness of sound, she is especially connected to musical enterprise. In fact, she is most often depicted holding an ancient Indian stringed instrument called a vinā. Sarasvatī represents the purity of mind required for inspiration to strike. Even on a cloudy day, the sun shines on regardless, above the clouds. And so, if we can learn to alight to a space beyond the clouds of our consciousness, we will find the light of inspiration, perpetually abiding. Inspiration is always there, it's just a question of receiving. And for this, the mud of our minds needs to be sufficiently pacified. Sarasvatī is the state of sattva—lightness, goodness. As such, the color white is sacred to Sarasvatī.

Sarasvatī's vehicle is the swan, the white, light bird that gracefully glides atop the surface of water. Swans are fabled to have the ability to separate milk from water when they're mixed together. They know the wheat from the chaff. Sarasvatī represents the highly refined consciousness that is capable of such discernment. The Sanskrit word for Swan in a modern context is haṃsa. *Due to the Sarasvatic symbolism ascribed to the haṃsa, great souls are called* parma-haṃsas, *great swans. This honorific title tells us that they have highly refined their discernment, and are of a very sattvic, pure nature. In a sense, they're embodiments of Sarasvatī.*

There's also an even more esoteric dimension to the word "haṃsa." In Indian sacred anatomy, there is a right, masculine energy channel and a left, feminine energy channel. These channels begin at the base of the subtle spine, in the root chakra, then weave up to meet again at the heart, and finally, at the third eye center. One who is fully realized is considered to have an opened third eye. The masculine solar channel is activated by the sacred sound "haṃ" and the feminine lunar channel is active by the word "sā." So, in the word haṃsa, the two channels meet at the third eye centre. When one is a "haṃsa" in this sense, the play of karma in this realm is completely illuminated by the light of consciousness, Sarasvatī herself. Remember Sarasvatī and all she represents while in this pose, as you strive to rise above the mud of life.

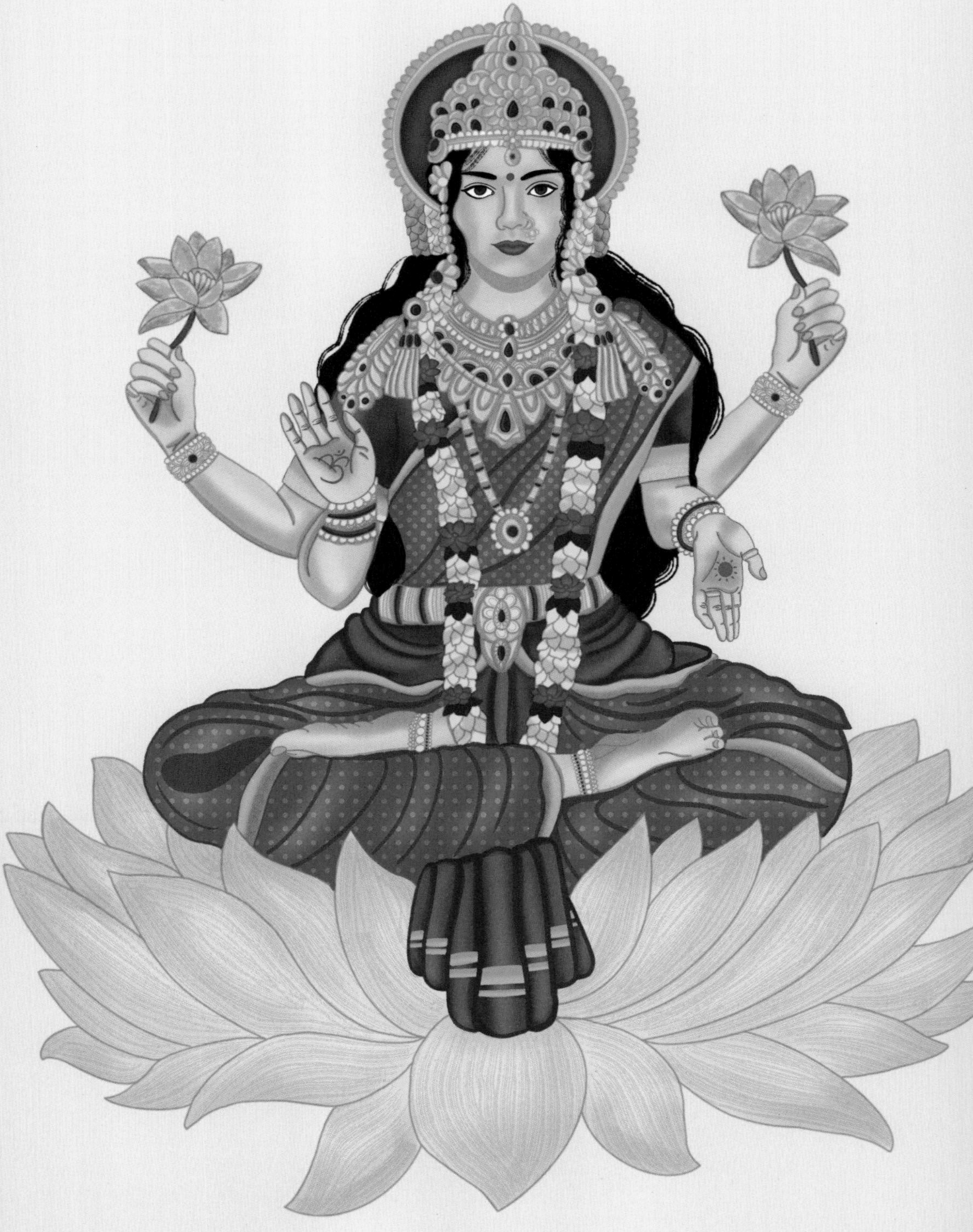

LOTUS POSE
PADMĀSANA

THE CHURNING OF THE COSMIC OCEAN (PART III)

THEMES
Transcendence
Purity
Poise

LONG AGO, THE DEMONS AND THE GODS had made a pact to churn the cosmic ocean in search of the Elixir of Immortality. The task was immense, but after several centuries of arduous work, the ocean began to produce great riches. First to emerge were the wish fullfilling cow, Kāmadhenu, given to the great sage Vasiṣṭha, and the great wish-fullfilling tree, Kalpa Vṛṣa, which was planted in the heavenly gardens of the gods. Then emerged the celestial nymph, Rambā, who henceforth lived among the Daityas. Next came 14 powerful gems, the 'pearls of the sea' most prominent of which was the Kaustubha stone. It was offered to Lord Viṣṇu, the great Preserver of the universe, who placed it at his heart. The entourage churned on.

After millennia of churning, and once the waters were crystal clear, a figure emerged from the Primordial oceans. It was the figure of the great Dhanvantari, celestial physician, born of the quest for immortality itself. As soon as his hands emerged from the blessed foam, a flash of light radiated from a vessel that he carried, and they knew at once that the nectar of immortality was therein. All were mesmerized by the brilliance of the vessel in which Dhanvantarī, carried the blessed Amṛta. A deep and weighty hush fell upon the scene, but this dignified moment was suddenly interrupted as the Daityas scrambled greedily to gain possession of the elixir.

Knowing the lustful nature of the Daityas, Viṣṇu transformed into his feminine form, the seductress Mohinī , mistress of infatuation. The demons were momentarily distracted from the elixir, and pursued Mohinī instead. As the beings of darkness chased the shadow of Viṣṇu, the Devas convened by the banks of the ocean to receive the sacred nectar. But to their surprise they noticed another form emerging form the primordial oceans, this time a feminine one, seated, floating upon a white lotus, and clothed resplendently in red cloth. In contrast to the illusory mistress of infatuation that Viṣṇu projected, this form was quite different. She was beautiful, authentic, and permanent. She was flanked by two elephants, Grace and Abundance, and the celestial musicians sang her praise as the cosmic oceans gave rise to her exquisite form. She was Lakṣmī, goddess of fertility, artistry, health, beauty, refinement, and abundance.

In two of her four hands, she carried celestial lotuses, representing transcendence from the mud of mundane existence. With her remaining hands, she gestured *abhaya mudra*, the "fear not" symbol, and *varada mudra*, signifying the conferring of gifts and good fortune. She was a mesmerizing sight. As the mistress of infatuation captivated the demons of darkness, so did Lakṣmī enthrall the beings of light, for she is light incarnate. Light knows no bounds, and so only when the universe was transformed to a state where it could hold immortality, only once the shadows were chased away, could the mother of light itself emerge.

Knowing her role as embodiment of divine love, Lakṣmī immediately sought to select a loving mate. After glancing at all of the assembled gods, she bowed before the waters and thanked them for her being. She understood that water is the locus of creativity and life; the ultimate source and symbol of purification, hydration, and sustenance for all things. From the waves emerged a beautiful garland, which she accepted as a token of her communion with the primordial ocean. She gazed into her own reflection in the water and understood her place in the universe. She knew that she was brought forth in tandem with immortality, and that she was the emissary of abundance. Like the boundless ocean, she transcended poverty, sickness, and solitude and thus brought with her the energy of prosperity, health, and love. Knowing her dharma, she walked past the assembly of gods until she was in the presence of the illustrious Viṣṇu, Preserver of the universe. To his supreme delight, she reverently garlanded him, speaking thus:

"I shall reside in your heart forevermore, O Glorious Lord, for no hearts assembled here are as vast. Your compassion is incomparable, Lord Viṣṇu! I am divine abundance, and can only dwell in a boundless space. And so, yours is the only heart wherein I may find a home. Your heart is all giving, and thus unencumbered by personal gain. Love is no mundane thing. My love for you shall be rendered boundless by your love for me, a love which we shall project onto eternity."

And so you have heard the story of the birth of Lakṣmī. Relish it. For your mind-stuff is the very primordial ocean of which the tale speaks, and you too, can—through tremendous upheaval—refine the layers of your consciousness to reveal the innate immortal purity that serves as the essence of your being. This essence is the ground of abundance. But you must neither ignore nor denounce your demons. They are an integral part of you. In order to acquire the most fruitful and balanced results, you must work with them. Abundance in all manifestations—fertility, prosperity, health, love—can be yours. And the lotus symbolizes all this.

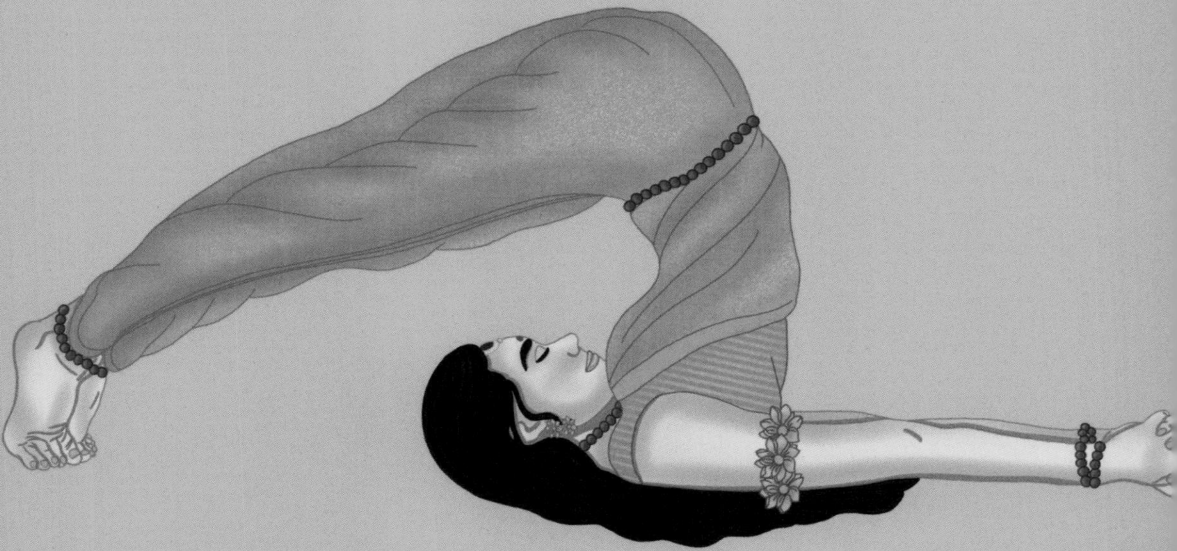

PLOUGH POSE
HALĀSANA

SĪTĀ, BORN OF THE EARTH

THEMES
Inversion
Balance
Endurance

Once, the great King Janaka was ploughing the fields around his palace as part of a sacred rite. It was springtime, and with spring blooms the fecundity of the earth. The more noble a king, the more bountiful the harvest within his kingdom. And so, accompanied by the Vedic priests, Janaka was ritually tilling the soil to appeal to Mother Earth, that she might bless the kingdom and bring forth bounty. At one point, Janaka's plough came to a standstill. He could not budge it. Concerned, he called to his attendant to remove the stone that blocked his way. The attendant bent down to rummage through the soil to find a large stone-lined basket. "Sire," said the attendant, "you best come see this for yourself." Janaka came round and picked up the basket, which was bedecked with jewels. He gently opened it and to his astonishment he found inside, a precious baby girl. "Mother Earth has given me the most bountiful harvest, even before I have sown! Glory to the goddess for sending me this child. I will raise her as my very own, and her name shall be Sītā." Janaka called for his wife, Sīradhvaja, and gave her the news. She was overjoyed since they were, as yet, childless. She cradled baby Sītā in her arms and carried her off to the palace to be raised as a princess.

Sītā grew up to be a beautiful, charming, noble young lady. She was the pride and joy of her parents. Time passed, and Sītā grew to marriageable age. The court advisors offered to invite bachelors from far and wide to be considered for the right to take her hand. Janaka, however, was quite protective of his dear daughter and would not consent to just anyone wedding this gift from the goddess, so he devised a strategy he was sure would separate the wheat from the chaff. Entrusted to his ancestors was Śiva's own Pināka bow, which had fallen from the heavens after a celestial battle. For generations, Janaka's line of succession had guarded the bow. It was so great, and so heavy, that no mere mortal could lift it, much less string it. So, Janaka decided that the suitor who would marry his daughter would be he who could string Śiva's bow!

Suitors came in great numbers to seek the hand of Sītā. Scores of gallant and handsome young men approached the Pināka bow to no avail. They couldn't even budge it, much less string it. Then it was Prince Rāma's turn. In one fell swoop, he raised and strung the bow, to the astonishment of all. Clearly destiny had meant for Rāma to marry Sītā, and marry they did. Sītā couldn't be happier. Janaka, too, was delighted to learn that Prince Rāma himself would have his darling Sītā's hand in marriage. Rāma and Sītā loved each other very much—so much so that when Rāma was exiled to the forest for 14 long years (due to the plotting of his stepmother), Sītā insisted on coming along. They roamed the lush woods having one great adventure after another, encountering sages, talking to monkeys, and many other marvelous things.

One day, in the woods, Sītā was abducted by the demon-king Rāvaṇa, and taken to his lair on the island of Laṅkā. After much effort, and with help from the monkey-people, Rāma was able to locate and rescue Sītā. He had been completely lost without her, and was so happy to have her back. Yet there was doubt among his forest assembly about Sītā's fidelity. After all, she had been with Rāvaṇa for an entire year. To lay the spiteful rumors to rest, Sītā summoned the sacred fire from the bowels of the earth as a testament to her purity. Fire burns away what isn't pure, so Sītā surrendered herself to grace and walked through the sacred flames. So pure was Sītā that not even a hair on her head was singed. Rāma embraced her, relieved.

But years later, once their exile was over and Rāma and Sītā had returned to rule, the gossip arose again in Rāma's kingdom. People can be quite petty, and gossiping about others can provide a welcome distraction from considering one's own flaws. The pernicious rumors became so widespread that Rāma's reign—and the stability of the realm itself—was threatened. So Rāma made an awful choice, and had his brother Lakṣmaṇa take Sītā out to a forest hermitage and leave her there. Sītā bemoaned her fate. She was pregnant with twins, and could not accept what had happened to her. She found solace in the ashram of the great sage Vālmīki, who comforted her and helped her raise her sons. Eventually, the boys learned the story of their father Rāma, and sought him out at his royal court to reconcile. But Sītā found no reconciliation in the world.

Once her sons had been accepted in the care of Rāma, Sītā bid farewell to sage Vālmīki and wandered out into the woods. In a sacred grove, she uttered a secret mantra, along with this prayer: "Mother Divine, Mother Earth, hear me, Sītā, your child. I've done what is right at every turn and yet, I've been abandoned, cast aside by the virtuous Rāma! How could this be? Why have you forsaken me?" Just then there was a rumbling in the earth, and the forest floor opened up. From it came an angelic voice: "Daughter, you are the child of my fecundity, born into the world to fullfill a purpose. You have now completed that purpose. Mortals can never attain happiness, so now that you have completed your mission among mortals, I call you to my bosom. I've supported you with every step you've taken. And you, like me, have endured the ills of man with forbearance and colossal strength. Return to me, child, where you belong, to merge with the rhythms of nature, and call forth the turning of the seasons. Return to your divine self!" And with this, the earth embraced Sītā. She was released from the burdens of her existence, and returned to the great Mother Earth.

As you practice plough pose, remember Sītā, born of Janaka's ritual ploughing. Remember the Rāmāyaṇa—the Tale of Rāma—as well as the Sītāyaṇa, the Tale of Sītā. Rāma is an avatāra *incarnation of the great god Viṣṇu who comes to Earth time and time again to restore dharma. Sītā was part of the divine plan, created so that Rāma would have occasion to defeat the great demon-king Rāvaṇa. But there is another tale to be told here. Sītā's is a story of inversions, where grace rises, born from the womb of Mother Earth. So pure is Sītā that fire cannot burn her. Hers is feminine power which endures all things, even the test of time. She is of the earth that endures all things and nurtures all creatures. Sītā's is a tale of the feminine divine, of the inherent divinity tied to nature and the fecundity of the earth. From earth was she born and to earth she returned, once her divine duty had been fullfilled.*

CRANE POSE
KRAUÑCĀSANA

SĪTĀ'S SEPARATION

THEMES
Poise
Majesty
Stature

ONCE, THE GREAT SAGE VĀLMĪKI posed the following question to the celestial figure Nārada: "Is there a man in the world who is truly virtuous, who is mighty yet knows the ways of righteousness?" To this, Nārada replied without hesitation that the great Prince Rāma possessed such virtues. Rāma was formidable in battle, yet wise and always true to his word. Nārada proceeded to tell Vālmīki the story of Rāma, of how he was cheated out of his throne and made to endure 14 long years of exile, of how his wife had been abducted by the demon-king Rāvaṇa, and how, with the help of the great monkey-men he waged a war, recovered Sītā, and returned to the capital Ayodhyā to rule at last. Vālmīki thanked Nārada for his fine exposition, and returned to his forest hermitage to ponder all Nārada had spoken of.

After some time, Vālmīki, with his pupil in attendance, went off to the riverbank to perform his morning ritual. It was a glorious day; the sun was shining upon the lush woods and Vālmīki was taking in the flora and fauna about him. After strolling for some time, he found a spot where the water ran clear and decided to take his ritual bath there. Near where he bathed, he spotted a pair of Sarus cranes, large, majestic colorful waterbirds who bond for life. The birds were engaging in their mating rituals. Vālmīki was admiring their beauty and capacity to love, when out of

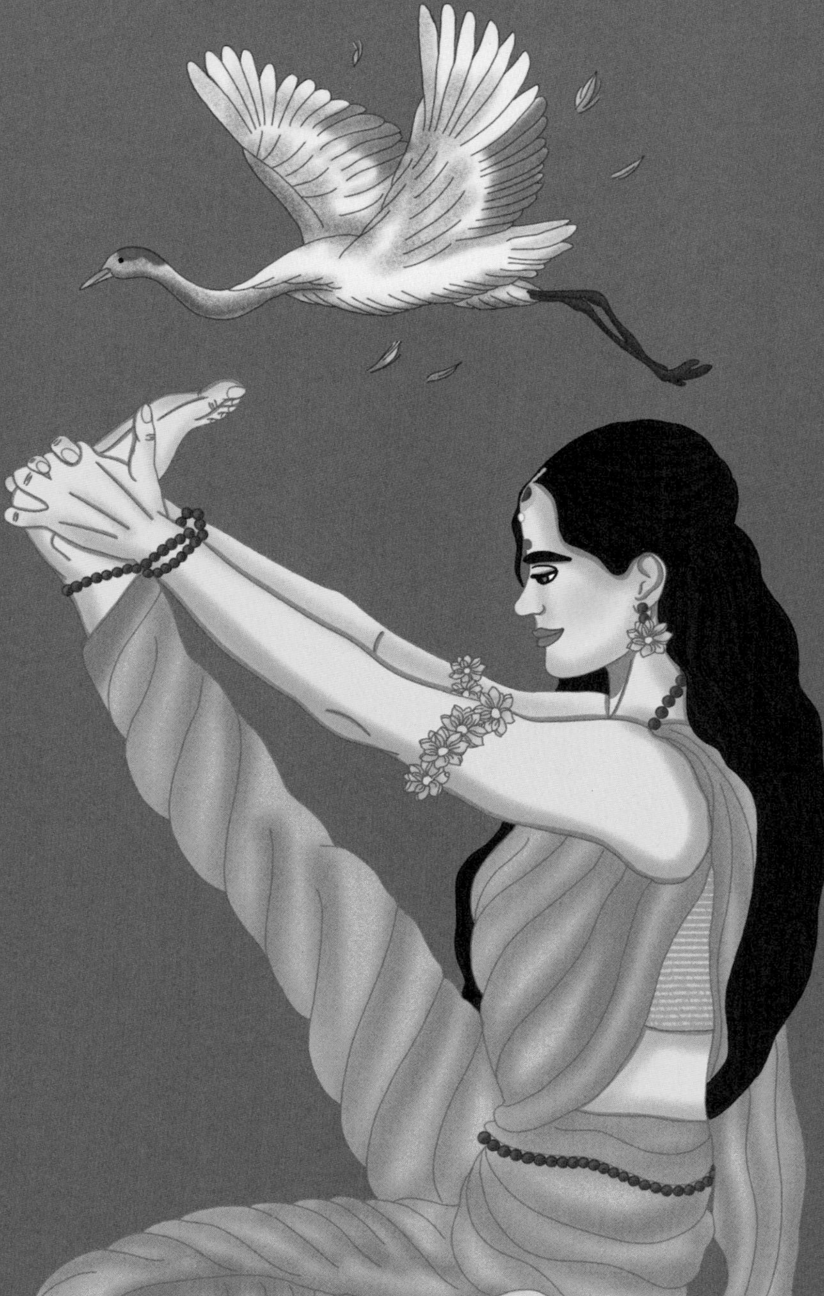

nowhere, a hunter's arrow pierced the scene, slaughtering the male of the pair. In shock and despair the female wailed for her fallen mate; a moment of tenderness eclipsed by senseless violence. The cry of the female Sarus caused great pity to well up in Vālmīki. With a tear in his eye, he turned to the vicious hunter and cursed him to soon die.

Both Vālmīki and his student were astonished, not so much at the destructive nature of Vālmīki's curse, but with the creative manner in which it was issued: cast in meter and rhyme. Upon being asked by his student what it was that he had uttered, Vālmīki declared that since it was born of śoka (grief), it would be called śloka (verse). Indeed, it was the first poetic verse ever spoken in the Sanskrit language. Vālmīki finished his bath, then went back to the ashram, deep in thought. He soon received a visit from none other than Lord Brahmā, the Creator himself, who gave him a special task. "Since you are now aware of the story of Rāma, and have discovered verse, you will write an epic, detailing the story of the great Rāma and his beloved wife Sītā." And so, Vālmīki set out to write the Rāmāyaṇa.

Vālmīki understood well why Lord Brahmā had allocated this task to him. He had been given the content by Nārada, had spontaneously invented the verse in the forest, but also, he had been moved by the tragic moment he had witnessed while bathing. He would need to remember this heartbroken feeling, for the story of Rāma and Sītā that he was to transcribe into poetic form was indeed a tragic tale of many separations. Not only were the two of them forced to endure 14 long years of exile in the forest, but while there, Sītā was abducted by the demon King Rāvaṇa. For a whole year, she dwelt, captive, at his court on the island of Laṅkā, and the two lovers in exile were separated even from each other.

With the help of the monkey god, Hanumān, and his people, Rāma was able to wage war upon Rāvaṇa and rescue her, but though Rāma and Sītā were overjoyed to be reunited, their separation had taken its toll, and things were never quite the same. Rāma expressed doubts about Sītā's purity since she had been held captive by another man for a year. Sītā, outraged, called forth the sacred fire and declared: "Fire burns away all that is impure. Surely the wise Rāma knows this. And so, I shall walk through the fire, and you will know by all that is burned away how much impurity is within me!" She walked through, completely unscathed, displaying her faithfulness and purity for all to see. Rāma was convinced, and relieved. But even this wasn't enough to quell the vicious rumors about her that were already spreading throughout the Kingdom.

Once their exile was over, and they returned to court to rule, the issue of the widespread gossip about Sītā's fidelity became unavoidable for Rāma, now King of Ayodhyā. Despite all Sītā had done to prove herself, and despite the fact that she was pregnant with twins, fathered by Rāma, he sent her away, to preserve the stability of his reign. Eventually she would seek solace at the very same ashram where this tale began, and be received by the great sage Vālmīki.

As you engage this elegant posture, reflect upon the majesty of the Sarus crane—its beauty, its grace, its capacity for courtship and love. The elongated leg is perhaps reminiscent of the arrow that struck the male of the pair before Vālmīki. But in your mood, you are relaxed and connected, like when the cranes were moving and singing together before the moment of sorrow arrived.

CRESCENT MOON POSE

AÑJANEYĀSANA

HANUMĀN'S FEMININE POWER

THEMES
Reverence
Devotion
Strength

LONG AGO, DEEP IN THE FORESTS of the Himālayan foothills, there dwelt the great race of monkey-people. Though they swung through branches and possessed long tails, they also belonged to an advanced culture. They were a great civilization of simian beings, hidden in the forests away from the world of men. They were called the Vānaras. One of their chieftains was named Kesarī and his wife was called Añjanā. Kesarī, would be away for weeks on end on hunting trips or expeditions, supporting neighboring clans, and in his absence, the tribe would turn to Añjanā for leadership. She was an extraordinarily powerful woman, the foundation of her community. Whether the task at hand required great skill in foraging, great strength to help the clan weather the fierce Himālayan storms, or the great courage and knowledge needed to safely deliver offspring, she could always be depended upon. Añjanā was also a great devotee of Lord Śiva. Daily she would chant his mantras, meditating on his form. She even had a sacred Lingam stone that she installed in her home, offering it fruit, flowers, milk, water, honey, and a variety of Śiva's preferred offerings. Sometimes she would worship Śiva from dusk until dawn, when her community duties began. Hers was a pure heart of unadulterated devotion to the lord. It was from him she drew her strength to be such a pillar of her community.

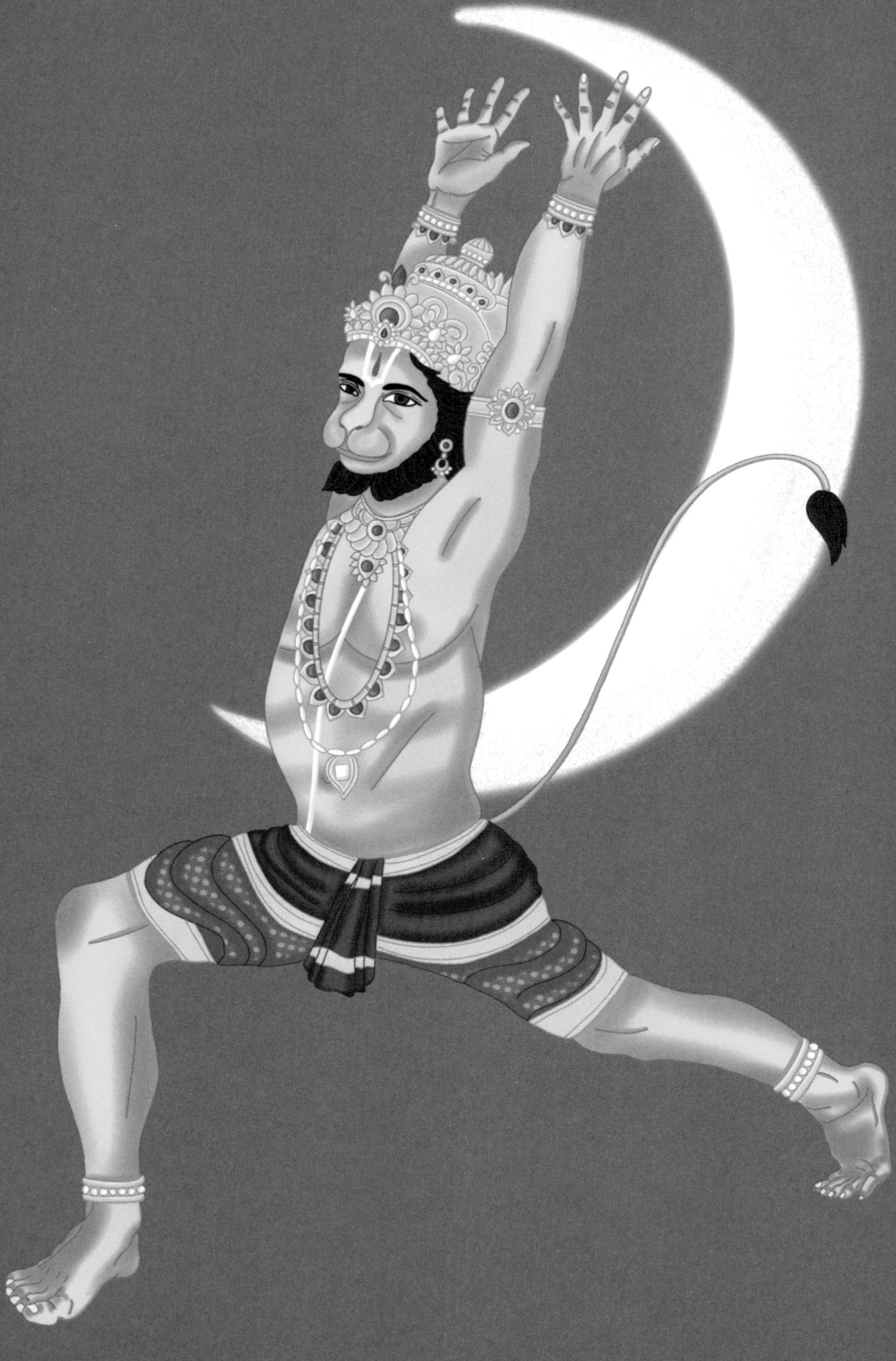

Añjanā had a full and fullfilling life, except in one domain. She and Kesarī were childless, after many years of trying. So, Añjanā decided to worship Lord Śiva with the express desire to conceive a child. For weeks, she held a vigil, worshipping the great Blue-Throated Lord day and night. Her prayers went straight to Lord Śiva, meditating in his mountain abode atop the Himālayas. The lord had been quite impressed and pleased with her incredible devotion over the years. He also admired the way in which she conducted herself in her community, offering support at every turn. Śiva thought to himself, "Since the selfless Añjanā has worshipped me, day in and day out, wanting nothing more than to please me, I will definitely grant her a boon, now that she worships me with a wish in mind." The lord wanted to bless Añjanā with a son, and not just any son, an incredibly powerful one with a great destiny ahead of him. He would grant her a son of his own. Śiva called on the wind god Vāyu, and the next time he and his beloved Pārvatī were communing, he spilt his seed to be carried by Vāyu to the foothills below to impregnate Añjanā. To her utter delight, Añjanā conceived.

Añjanā gave birth to a wise, powerful, noble monkey-man named Hanumān. Hanumān was, at the same time, the son of the chieftain Kesarī, the son of Śiva, and the son of Vāyu, the wind god. But he only had one mother: Añjanā. His favorite epithet was Añjaneya, which means son of Añjanā. He loved his mother dearly, and learned a great deal from her; her devotion and strength set an invaluable example for him to emulate, and she also often shared lessons of profound wisdom with him. In one such moment, she asked him which was stronger, water or rock? Hanumān, of course, chose the rock. Añjanā then gave this teaching: "That's what most think, my son. Rock is masculine and water is feminine. The masculine appears stronger in the outer world. But the strength of the feminine comes from within. A stone axe cannot penetrate the tiny cracks the way water can. And even a great boulder can be split open by water flowing gently through its cracks, given time. You are a great and powerful warrior without question, but your true power will come from within, from devotion, surrender, sacrifice, and service to something greater, just as water, because it is soft and yielding, has strength enough to dissolve mountains," Hanumān was awed by the wisdom with which his mother gifted him.

Hanumān indeed proved himself to be most powerful as a warrior. Kesarī was proud of his son's colossal strength and martial prowess. None could best Hanumān, not monkey, human, or demon. Añjanā, on the other hand, was much prouder of the profound devotion she saw growing within him. She knew he had a great destiny, and that everything she taught him would be part of it. Hanumān did indeed become the greatest devotee of Rāma, incarnation of Viṣṇu, and his consort Sītā. He showed Rāma the same unadulterated devotion that Añjanā showed Śiva. Hanumān's true strength came from the inner world, through his spiritual connection to the divine. He never married, and remained ever chaste, sublimating his libidinal urges in pursuit of greater heights of psychic power. His upright tail represents the raised spiritual power that afforded him the ability to fly and to make himself much larger and smaller at will. Kuṇḍalinī is feminine, so those who wield it wield feminine power, derived from the inner world. Hanumān, of course, comingled this feminine power with masculine, martial outer power. On one occasion, Rāma's beloved brother Lakṣamaṇa fell ill and the only herb that could cure him was atop a faraway mountain. Hanumān flew to the mountain, but was unable to discern which herb was the right one. But not to be discouraged, he simply brought back the entire mountain. His colossal masculine strength here is powered by his feminine ability to surrender and serve something greater. The mountain was lifted by devotion. The example of inner strength and feminine power we see in Hanumān very much stems from him following the example of his extraordinary mother Añjanā.

Remember Hanumān and his maternal influence when doing crescent moon pose. Embody a spirit of surrender, reverence, and devotion. Interestingly, this pose is commonly found in Sūrya Namaskāra, which is a heating yoga sequence focused on activating solar, masculine energy in the body. Despite this, one adopts a mode of receiving and reverence when doing this sequence. The feminine and masculine work in tandem, and their essence runs far deeper than biology or sociology. These two principles inhabit all people, and the work of yoga is concerned with bringing them into balance.

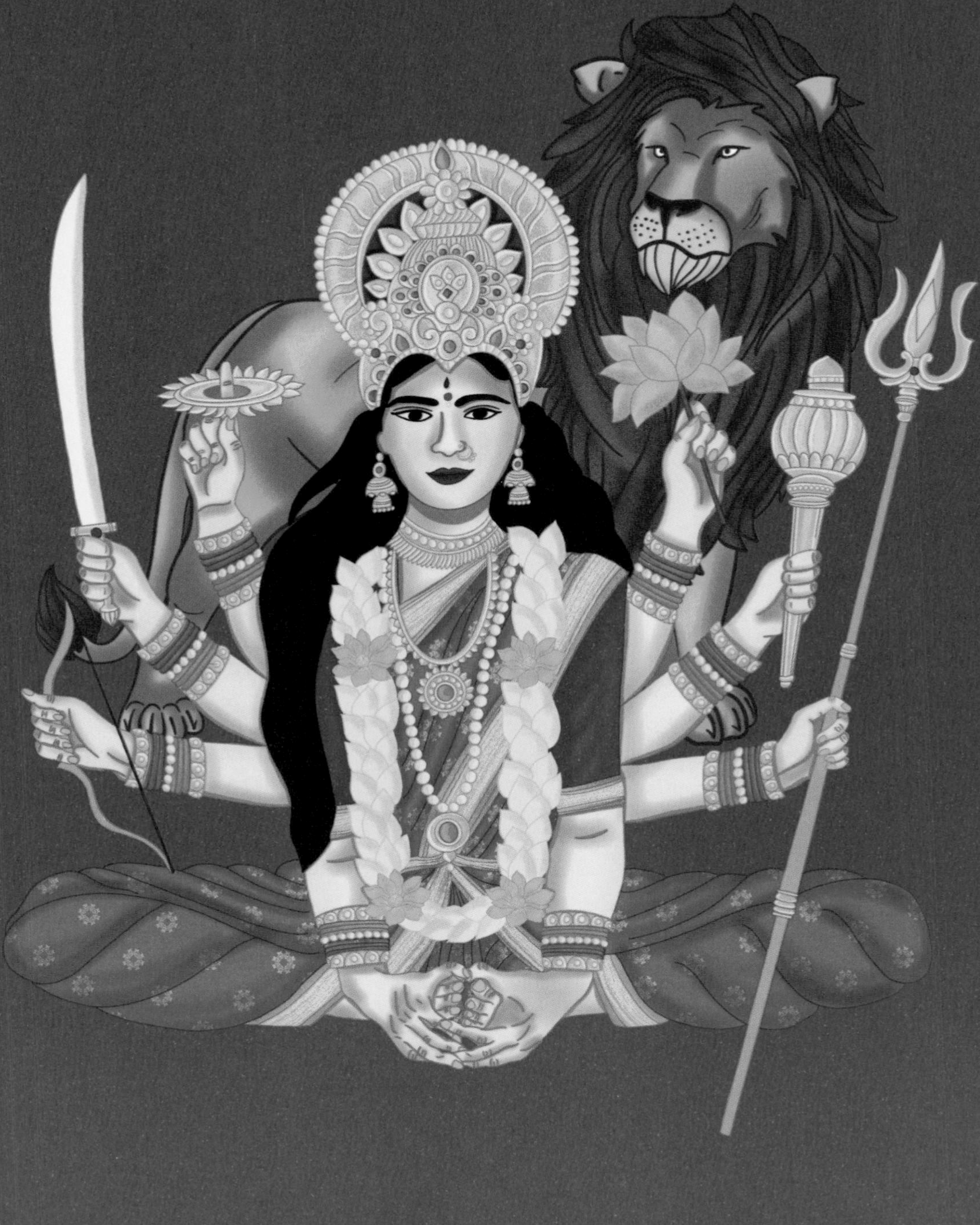

THRONE POSE
BHADRĀSANA

DURGĀ,
DIVINE QUEEN

THEMES
Poise
Power
Humility

ONCE THERE WAS A WISE AND NOBLE KING named Suratha, who treated his subjects as his own kith and kin. The kingdom prospered under his rule, until power-thirsty lords from adjoining lands began to usurp his domain. He retreated to his capital city, but even there, he was robbed of his dominion through the plotting of wicked ministers. Stripped of his power, beside himself with grief, he took to his horse and entered the deep dark forest to process what had happened. While there, he came across the hermitage of the great sage Medhas. So steeped in the principles of truth and compassion was the sage, that the wild beasts of the forest were tamed by his very presence. And so, the king found great solace in the hermitage, enjoying the peace there, and the melodious chanting of the sage and his students. Yet after some time, despair crept back into his mind.

The king was lamenting to himself in the vicinity of the ashram. Dejected, he wondered after the welfare of his citizens, his capital city, his pet elephant, his treasury, and all else that he had loved and lost. Right then, a lone merchant crossed his path, looking equally demoralized. The king greeted the merchant with kindness, asking after his woes. The merchant said that his own family had stolen his great wealth and cast him out of his home, to wander as a beggar.

"But I can't help but wonder," concluded the merchant, "how my wife and sons are keeping. Are they eating properly? Are the boys doing their homework?" The merchant sighed in despair and concern after the welfare of his loved ones.

"How can you possibly be so attached to people who treated you so cruelly?" asked the king.

"Indeed," said the merchant. "I know better, but can't help myself."

"Well, we're not so different you and I," said the king. "Just as you came by, I was lamenting my own affairs, attached to my kingdom, court, and subjects. You and I are the blind leading the blind! Perhaps we should seek the counsel of the wise sage, Medhas, whose hermitage this is." The two dejected men approached the sage with respect and humility, asking if he could shed light on their attached natures.

"Well, noble king," began the sage, "this is a simple thing. All creatures are attached. We live in this world under the illusion of separation, propelled by attachment to those we care about. Desire is the seed of creation. We are all part of this great matrix of life, under the spell of the great goddess Mother Māyā who deludes all beings. But Mother Māyā is also Mother Wisdom, both which are aspects of the formidable Mother Durga! She may delude you with the play of the world, but she can just as easily remove the veil. She is the source of all power, the Lady of Lords, Queen of Kings, sovereignty itself!" Mesmerized, the king requested to know more.

The sage told them three tales expounding the greatness of the goddess. First, he spoke of how she was called on by the Creator himself at the dawn of time to save creation from the demons Madhu and Kaiṭabha. He then proceeded to tell the tale of how the goddess restored the power of Indra and the gods when they were usurped by the great buffalo demon Mahiṣa. Lastly, he told the tale of the cataclysmic battle of the goddess and her forces (including Kālī and the Seven Mothers) against the demonic duo, Śumbha and Niśumbha, when they usurped the throne of Indra. "And so," concluded the sage, "by the great goddess are you and this merchant deluded, and it is by her grace you can be freed. She is the source of all power in the universe, the power of māyā and the power of wisdom. Take refuge in her, worship her, and your desires will be fullfilled."

The merchant and the king took leave of the wise sage, expressing their gratitude for his teachings. They made their way to a riverbank and crafted a clay icon of the goddess, which they consecrated with Sanskrit mantras. They then worshipped her day and night with water, incense, fruits, flowers, and flame. For three long years they worshipped her, chanting her sacred hymns, meditating on her glories and her divine form. Pleased by their penance, the goddess appeared before them and granted them each a boon of their choosing. The merchant humbly asked her for the supreme knowledge that results in transcendence of "I-ness" and "my-ness." He sought liberation from material creation. The king, on the other hand, wished for the return of his kingdom.

"Wise merchant, you shall have the boon you seek: you will be liberated from the cycle of rebirth by my divine grace. And you, noble king, will receive your boon also: in three days' time you will confront your enemies, and through my grace, you will be victorious and regain your kingdom. It will be yours for the rest of your days. Then once you have completed this incarnation, I will exalt you to be reborn as the next Manu, Lord of the Age, progenitor of all humanity, reborn as the son of the sun." Delighted, they prostrated before her, singing her praises as she vanished. And so it came to pass that by the grace of the goddess, a merchant gained spiritual liberation, and a deposed king not only regained his throne, but was rewarded for his care for the world, and became Manu of the next age.

The world is the very body of the great goddess. Hers is the work of kings in that she safeguards the collective welfare on the heavenly sphere, just as the king does here on Earth. Enlightenment and illusion, mokṣa and māyā, both are divine, for without the world of separation, name and form, souls could not exhaust their karmas and learn their lessons. Although the goddess is regal, and safeguards the throne of Indra and earthly kings like Suratha, she does not herself occupy a throne. Above and beyond being a sovereign, she is sovereignty itself. The great kings in these tales draw their royal authority from the wellspring of power that is the Mother Divine, source of all things. Remember this as you engage this pose, with poise, power, and humility before the greatness of the goddess.

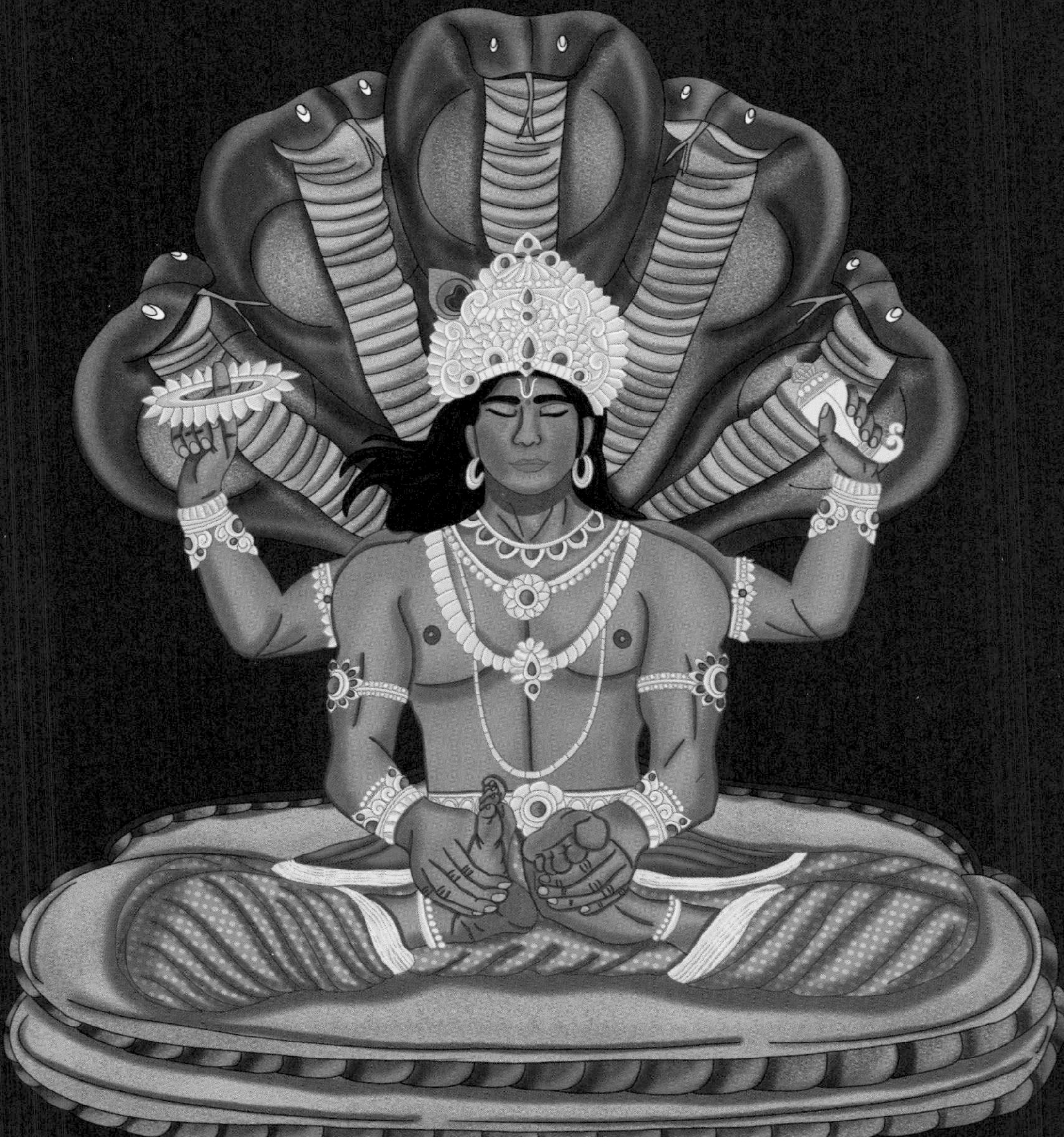

NAVEL POSE
KANDĀSANA

THE GODDESS SAVES CREATION

THEMES
Strength
Poise
Courage

JUST AS THE DAWN FOLLOWS DUSK, so too does the dawn of creation follow the dusk of the last. At the end of the previous age, Śiva had performed his rapturous dance of destruction, and dissolved all things into the primordial oceans. For the universe is fundamentally without beginning and without end, ceaselessly engaged in cycles of cosmic creation, preservation, and destruction. In the electric silence before the dawn of time, the Lord Viṣṇu lay sleeping on his serpent couch, floating upon the endless ocean. He would not wake again until he was needed. Viṣṇu is the great Preserver, now simply waiting for Brahmā, to create the universe anew.

From slumbering Viṣṇu's divine navel emerged a celestial lotus in which Brahmā, the Creator himself, was born. He opened his eyes and beheld the glorious scene about him. Beyond the root of the divine lotus in which he was situated, he beheld the body of Viṣṇu sprawled out before him. Beyond that, lay the oceanic abyss. Brahmā gazed out upon it and focused his mind, preparing to create all things. He took a deep inbreath and was about to shatter the silence with a resounding cosmic "OṂ", when he noticed something quite unexpected. Out of Viṣṇu's right ear had emerged a demon, Madhu! Then out of his left ear emerged another demon, Kaiṭabha! The demons made a mad dash across the body of the lord, intent on destruction. They planned to uproot Brahmā's lotus and destroy creation, even before it was created!

Brahmā was panicked. His was a creative task, and he possessed no weapons. He shook the stem of the divine lotus in hopes of waking Viṣṇu to warn him about the approaching assault, but Viṣṇu could not be awakened! He was sound asleep in his yogic slumber. So, Brahmā gathered himself, took a deep breath, and turned inwards for inspiration. Even the gods themselves are but pieces of the cosmic puzzle: none have the whole picture. Brahmā connected to the source for inspiration, and inspiration he received. He channelled a divine hymn to the Great Mother, and recited it aloud. In the hymn, he praised the Mother as the source of all things, as the power behind creation, preservation, and destruction. He honored her as the aspect of creation that deludes all creatures, as Mother Māyā herself, knowing that illusion and enlightenment are two sides of the same coin. Pleased by this praise, the Mother released her grasp on Viṣṇu and he became fully awake.

Viṣṇu immediately sprang to his feet, knowing what he must do, and engaged the demons in combat. He swirled around in the primordial oceans, battling the demons which had emerged from his own ears with his divine discus. Centuries went by as the battle ensued. Seeing the stalemate, the Mother decided to tip the scales of destiny in Viṣṇu's favor. So, she used her powers of illusion on Madhu and Kaiṭabha, and they became completely deluded by their own power. All things operate by the grace of the Mother's divine power, and when beings misapprehend it as their own, their egos are fed. Power deludes when one can't see its actual source: the divine. And so, deluded and feeling quite satisfied with themselves, the demons decided to taunt Viṣṇu with a show of their power.

"Viṣṇu, you pathetic excuse for a god! Here you are, unable to defeat two demons that have grown from the wax of your own ears! What kind of god are you, so weak, so powerless? We are far more powerful than you, since two is better than one! We're so much more powerful that we'll grant you a boon, pathetic Viṣṇu!"

Normally Viṣṇu would have been outraged at the utter insolence of Madhu and Kaiṭabha. But, having been fully released from the grasp of Mother Māyā, he was completely awake and seeing clearly. When we see the play of māyā, we are not trapped by the ill intent of the other. We understand that things aren't happening "to" us, but "for us." So, blessed with the wisdom to see beyond the play of Mother Māyā, Viṣṇu was without ego. He graciously accepted their insolent offer: "So be it, powerful Madhu and Kaiṭabha, I accept your offer!"

Pleased with themselves, and drunk with Viṣṇu's apparent acquiescence, they proceeded along their path: "Anything you want! We are truly powerful! Just name your boon, fallen god, and out of pity we will grant it to you!"

"Well my boon is that I should be able to kill you!"

Thinking themselves clever, the demons replied, "Being honorable beings, we will honor our boon. You may kill us anywhere in this primordial ocean where there is no water!"

Viṣṇu agreed, and swiftly swooped them up above the oceanic abyss, where he severed them in two with his discus. And that was the end of the demons.

The waters were quelled and, by the grace of Mother Māyā, Viṣṇu returned to his yogic slumber. Brahmā again emerged from the celestial lotus and beheld the wonderous sight before him. But this time his awe was augmented by what he had learned. Trials and tribulations carry with them great lessons indeed. This time, as he called forth cosmic sound and created all things, as he manifested the galaxies, planets, and stars, he was all too conscious of the fact that he was merely an instrument of the great goddess, Mother Power, who energizes all things. His power to create was a portion of Mother Power's power, as was Viṣṇu's power to preserve, and Śiva's power to destroy. And this is how the Creator became aware of the presence of Mother Māyā, whose grace powers all creation.

This myth is rich with the mechanics of self-actualization. Consider each character as aspects of self. You are the sleeping Viṣṇu, imperilled by demons of your own unconscious, threatening to sabotage what you wish to manifest. Brahmā is your creative capacity, your ability to produce, create, and manifest the life you want. And, of course, the goddess is that divine power all about us, which we can summon and channel for the sake of battling our demons and actualizing the life we desire. Just as Brahmā is born of the navel of Viṣṇu, so, too, does your sacred center of manifestation (your manipūra chakra) reside within your navel region. When you feel powerless, you may well feel a sinking feeling in the "pit of your stomach." This posture brings active awareness to your subtle navel, which is the seat of fire in the body. You activate and stoke that fire so that you can dispel your fears and courageously combat your demons, inner and outer. This will put you in good stead to create the universe you desire.

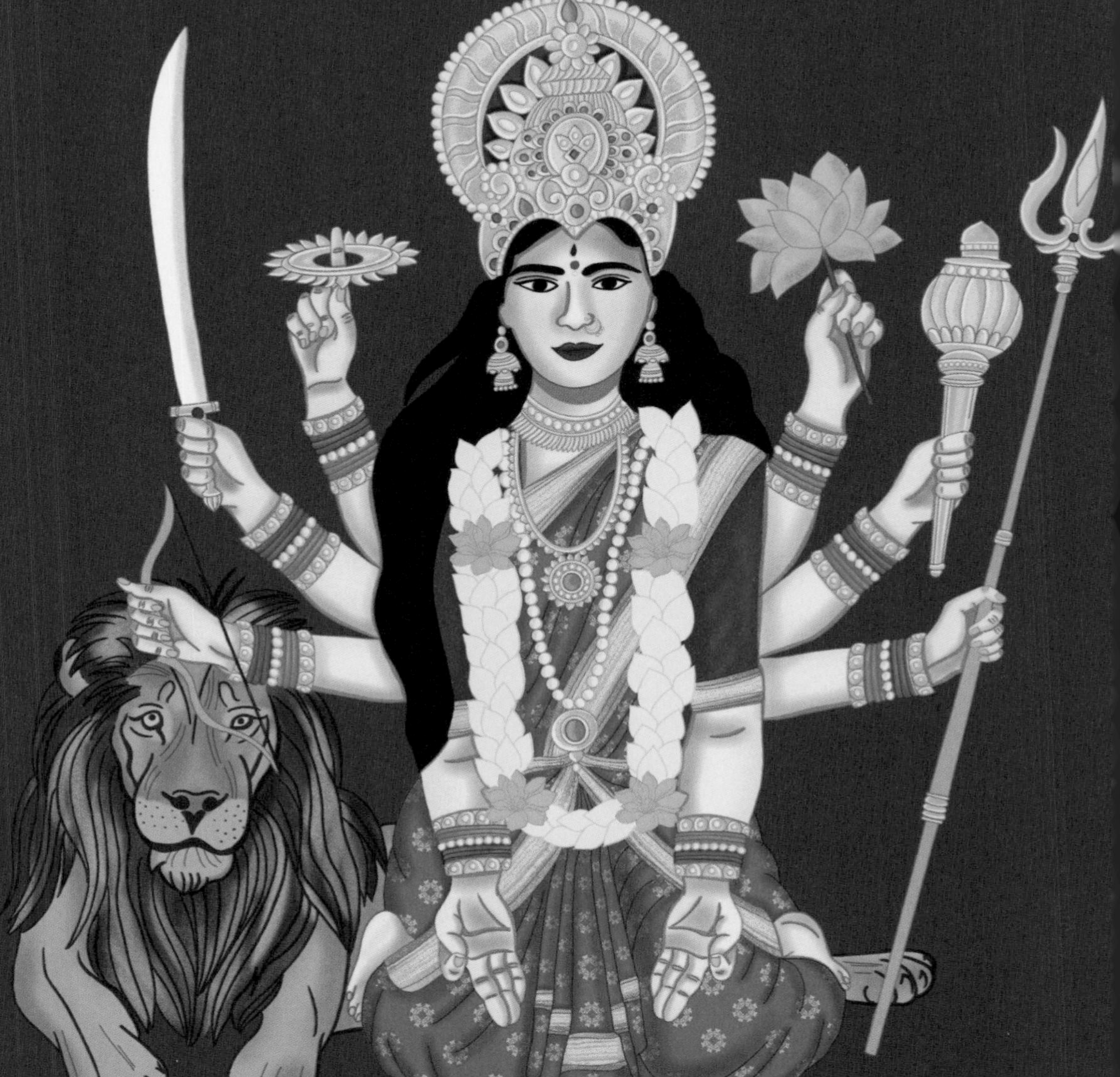

HERO POSE
VĪRĀSANA

DURGĀ, DIVINE MOTHER AND DIVINE WARRIOR

THEMES
Poise
Power
Containment

ONCE, THE SHAPESHIFTING BUFFALO demon, Mahiṣa, had usurped the throne of heaven, casting Indra and the gods out of paradise to wander the earth as mere mortals. The gods were robbed of their rightful status, their riches, and their share of the sacrifices. They were displaced and demoralized, roaming the earth and wondering what to do. Indra, wielder of the great thunderbolt, led his entourage of deposed gods to the great god Viṣṇu, the cosmic Preserver, to seek his advice. Unsure as to how to defeat the buffalo demon, Viṣṇu led Indra and the gods to the abode of Brahmā, the Creator. Four-headed Grandfather Brahmā was engaged in his cosmic meditations upon their arrival. Upon being presented with the situation, Brahmā scratched his heads and thought for a moment before suggesting they pay Śiva the Destroyer a visit. So, the entire entourage of Indra and the gods, Viṣṇu, and Brahmā all made their way to the abode of Śiva in the Himālayas and presented their situation.

Upon hearing the predicament of the gods, Śiva was outraged that Mahiṣa would dare usurp the throne of heaven. He scowled in indignation at the shapeshifting demon's audacity, his face contorted with rage. From his deeply furrowed brow, a beam of fiery light emerged. At this, Viṣṇu, too, became outraged, as did Brahmā, and shafts of light were emitted from them as well. The outrage of Indra and the gods, too, resulted in rays of light being emitted from their bodies. All the radiant beams converged as one, the size of a mountain, blazing with a furious incandescence. The cosmic beams pervaded the heavens and were emitted in all directions. The light coalesced into a majestic being. The gods witnessed the formation of a radiant feminine form right before their eyes. It was Durgā, the great goddess, mother of existence.

The energy emitted from each of the gods formed a different part of the great goddess. From Śiva's light was formed her face, Yama's her hair, Viṣṇu's her arms. The moon god's soft radiance formed her breasts, and from Indra's light her waist was forged. The fire god's light became her eyes, her eyebrows formed from dawn and dusk, and the wind became her ears. And so, the light of the gods of heaven converged to manifest the goddess, mother of the universe. The gods rejoiced at the appearance of the divine Mother, knowing she would fullfill their wishes and restore their power.

The gods then cloned their weapons to present to the goddess. Śiva bestowed a trident, Viṣṇu a discus and conch, Agni (the god of fire) a spear, Vāyu (the god of wind) a bow and an inexhaustible quiver of arrows. Viśvakarman, the divine craftsman, gave her an axe and impenetrable armor. Yama (the god of death) presented her a staff, Kāla (the god of time) a sword and shining shield, Varuṇa (the god of the waters) a noose, and the Creator Brahmā gave her prayer beads. She even received a thunderbolt from Indra (the god of storms.)

Sūrya the sun god poured his brilliance into her pores, and the celestial oceans produced pearls, wonderous garments, earrings, bracelets, anklets, and all manner of radiant adornments, including, a magnificent lotus to grace one of her many hands. The Himālayas gave the goddess a majestic lion mount to ride. So it was, that the cosmic mother was manifested by the outrage of the gods, and honored and adorned in their hour of need. The glorious goddess accepted their offerings and rode into battle, her defiant laughter resounding throughout the world. The gods exclaimed, "Victory! Jaya Jaya!" as she set out to reconquer heaven's throne.

She manifested hordes of her own to engage Mahiṣa's evil forces. Her roar filled the heavens, and the earth shook as the great battle began. Swords, missiles, and arrows flew in all directions as the armies clashed upon the field. Though Mahiṣa's hordes engaged them with javelins, swords, nooses, axes, and all manner of weapons, the Devī's forces prevailed and the demonic forces were overcome. Then Mahiṣa, the great buffalo demon, rode into battle to engage the Devī himself. The Earth quaked under his great hooves as he flung mountains aside with his fearsome horns. His mighty bellows filled the air and his tail lashed the oceans into a frenzy. His power was great and terrible, and the ousted gods were stricken with fear as they looked on. He made a mad rush at the goddess. Enraged, she bound him with her noose, but he turned himself into a lion and escaped. She then decapitated the lion, but not soon enough for him to emerge in his human form, sword in hand. As the goddess pummeled him with arrows, he shapeshifted again into his elephant form. Though the goddess ran him through with her sword, he shifted again to his buffalo form.

The goddess, though mad with anger, was not discouraged. She drank a celestial brew, her eyes reddened, and she laughed again and again. The demon met the din with bellows of his own. Inebriated with the divine brew, the goddess exclaimed, "Go ahead and bellow, fool! Your braying will be replaced with the cheering of the gods as I slay you where you stand!" With these words, she leapt upon the shapeshifting buffalo overlord, pinned him down beneath her feet, and beheaded him with her sword once and for all. The gods rejoiced at the triumph of the goddess, who had accomplished this great task that no one else could. Every one of them praised her majesty and might from the depths of their being, bowing deeply in heartfelt reverence. Pleased by their praise, she offered the gods a boon of their choosing. They asked her to return in future when, in great need, they may call upon her again. Granting their boon, the goddess vanished, having restored the power of the gods.

While there are a great many heroes to draw on for inspiration from the world of Indian mythology, the story of the manifestation of Durgā is apt indeed. It speaks to the strength of the feminine power that emerges from harmonious cooperation. Durgā emerges from the collective outrage of the gods. And when her task is accomplished, she vanishes. She does not occupy the throne, but safeguards it for the gods. In this pose one does not strut like a peacock, but sits like a lion who has nothing to prove and feels the power established within. In hero pose, you straighten your spine and inwardly activate your core. You stand to attention as a great warrior, poised, powerful, and contained.

SCORPION POSE
VṚŚCIKĀSANA

KĀLĪ AND THE SCORPION'S STING

THEMES
Strength
Intensity
Focus

LONG AGO, TWO DEMONS, Śumbha and his brother Niśumbha, waged war upon the gods of heaven, and succeeded in usurping Indra's throne. The gods were left to roam the earth as mere mortals. It was not the first time they had suffered this fate. There was once a time before, when the great buffalo demon Mahiṣa had usurped heaven's throne, and in their collective outrage they had summoned forth the great goddess, mother of existence. The goddess battled Mahiṣa and restored the sovereignty of the gods. Thereupon, Indra and the gods, bodies bent in reverence and hearts filled with gratitude, raised their voices in glorious praise to the goddess. Pleased by this, she granted them a boon of their choosing. Since their wishes had already been fullfilled by the destruction of Mahiṣa and restoration of their sovereignty, they wished that the goddess would return in future whenever they remembered her. And so, now cast out of heaven once again by the wicked Śumbha and Niśumbha, they set out to summon the goddess in their time of need.

The gods went up to the highest mountain peaks, and again raised their voices in collective praise to the glory of the goddess. They hailed her as the power within all living beings, comprising their natural impulses and their virtues. The hailed the holy goddess as the power of sleep, hunger, thirst, beauty, faith, peace, and prosperity. Pleased by their praise,

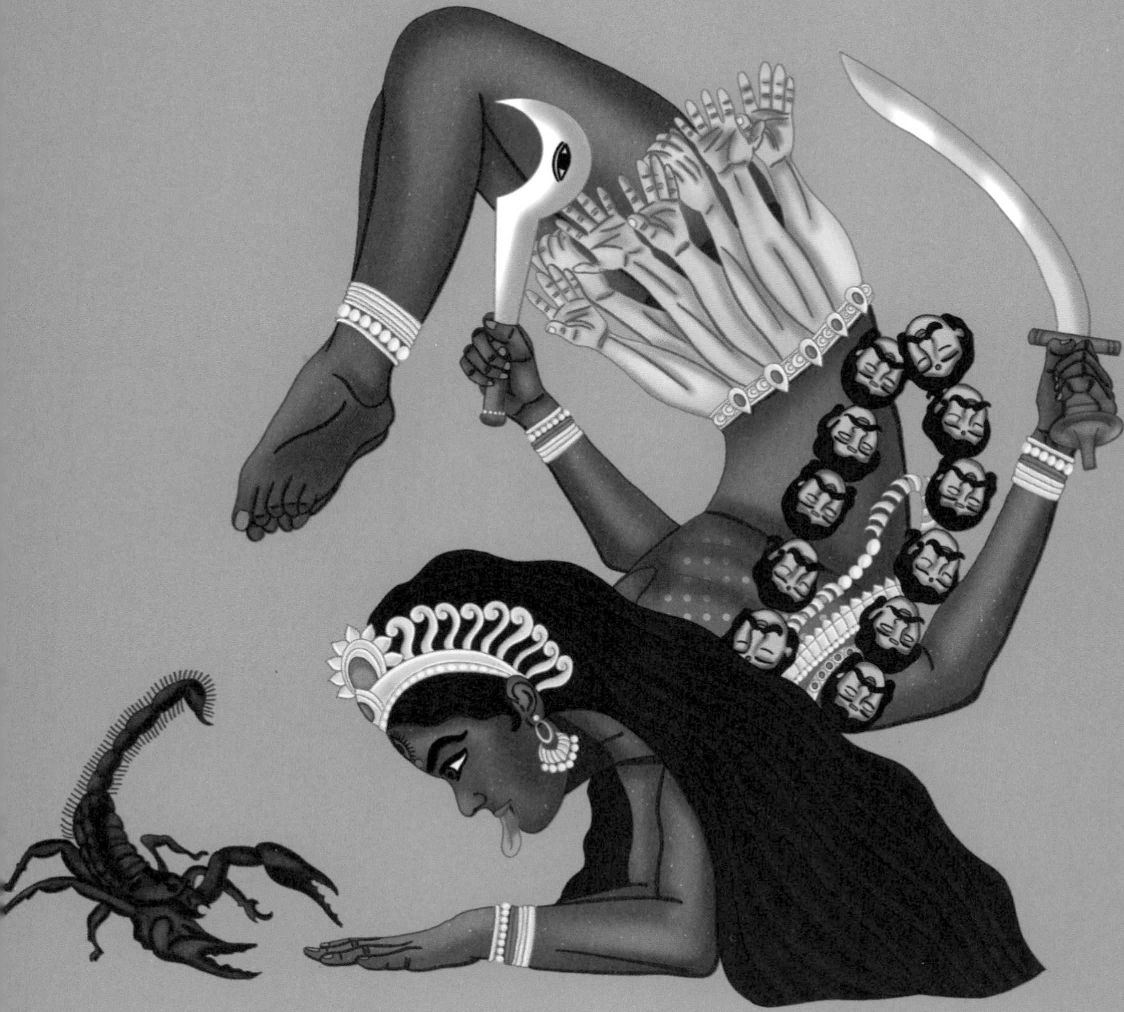

the goddess again manifested before them. She was resplendent upon her lion mount, her radiance lighting up the mountainside. The demons, Caṇḍa and Muṇḍa, servants of Śumbha and Niśumbha, happened to be nearby, and were utterly captivated by the beauty of the goddess. They rushed back to their demon overlord with the following report: "Masters, we have come across the most beautiful of women in the mountains. Nowhere has such beauty been seen. You should find out who she is and take possession of her. She casts her radiance in all directions, a true jewel among women. Since you have already acquired the greatest jewels, elephants, horses, and all the greatest riches of the heavens and the earth, it's only fitting you take ownership of this prize among women at once!" And so, the demons dispatched a messenger to the goddess to relay their position.

The messenger approached the goddess saying, "I am the messenger of Śumbha, king of the demons, and supreme sovereign of earth and heaven. He sends the message that since all of the world belongs to him, and all of its finest jewels, then so too should you, O precious gem among women. You shall accompany us to my master's abode, and become his wife." Playing into their delusion, the goddess batted her eyelashes and coquettishly proclaimed that she had made a foolish vow when she was young, and that the only man she would marry would be he who could best her in battle. Despite the messenger's protests that she wouldn't stand a chance, she insisted that he take the message back to Śumbha.

Outraged at such a response, Śumbha sent forth his general, Dhūmralocana, and his army, proclaiming that either the goddess would accept his proposal willingly, or else be dragged by her hair back to him, against her will. Upon being presented with the ultimatum, the goddess said to Dhūmralocana, "Well, if you and your powerful forces wish to drag me by my hair, what can a lone woman like me possibly do? Proceed as you must." With this, Dhūmralocana made a move to drag her by her hair, but before he could reach her, she let out a wrathful outcry that reduced him to ashes. Her lion mount ripped apart his army without mercy or hesitation. When news of this reached Śumbha, he dispatched Caṇḍa and Muṇḍa themselves, along with an even bigger army, to drag her forcibly back to become his wife. As the demon forces approached the goddess, she was smiling contently, resplendent upon the mountainside. They made a dash to grab her, but she let out another angry cry. Her face turned black as ink with wrath, and from her outraged, knitted brow sprang forth the goddess Kālī, a manifestation of the mother's power.

Kālī was dreadful to behold, armed with sword and noose, and adorned with a garland of severed heads. She was emaciated, her body like that of a scorpion, with lolling tongue, sunken eyes, and a cackle that filled the four directions. Kālī sprang forth to singlehandedly battle the army. She seized some by the hair and some by the neck, while others she pulverized underfoot. She caught their missiles in her mouth, grinding them between her teeth. Kālī ravaged the enemy forces in one fell swoop. She then severed the heads of Caṇḍa and Muṇḍa and brought them back to the goddess as a present, saying, "Here are the heads who could not see straight even with four eyes. I present them to you as a trophy of our triumph!" Pleased by the prowess of Kālī, the goddess declared, "Since you have fetched me the heads of the vile Caṇḍa and Muṇḍa, you will be hailed from this day forth as the goddess Cāmuṇḍa!"

The goddess Cāmuṇḍa is connected with the scorpion. Both are able to sting in times of defense. So, as you do this pose representing the scorpion about to sting, remember the role of Kālī in destroying Caṇḍa and Muṇḍa. While nonviolent compassion is indeed the crown jewel of Indian philosophy, let us not forget that there is a time for peace and a time for war. Reason would not work with foes such as those found in this story. Such forces intent on discontent and destruction can only be stopped with force. Remember, it was the demons who threatened, and then attempted to force their will upon the goddess, objectifying and commodifying her as something to be owned by the demon overlord Śumbha. It's clear that they acted from a place of utter delusion. Barring all other means, the scorpion's sting is necessary to paralyze such destructive forces.

LEG BEHIND HEAD POSE

EKA-PĀDA-ŚĪRŚĀSANA

DIVINE DECAPITATION

THEMES
Sacrifice
Surrender
Centeredness

LONG AGO, THE DEMON BROTHERS Śumbha and Niśumbha had usurped the throne of heaven, casting out Indra and the gods to wander the earth as mere mortals. The gods, at first, weren't sure what to do, but then they remembered a boon they had received previously from the great goddess, who promised she would return in times of distress, whenever they called her to mind. So, they went up to the highest peaks of the Himālayan mountains and hymned the glories of the goddess. The goddess appeared, resplendent, and the gods rejoiced at her manifestation, knowing only she could restore their power.

Caṇḍa and Muṇḍa, the demon minions of Śumbha, were lurking in the vicinity and chanced upon the goddess. They were completely taken by her radiance, and ran back to report what they saw to their master, suggesting he claim her for himself. So, Śumbha dispatched a messenger to the goddess, demanding that she become his wife. He owned all of the greatest jewels in the world, and so he should take possession, he thought, of this greatest jewel among women. Upon hearing this, the goddess smiled and informed the messenger that she had long ago vowed that only he who defeated her in battle could become her husband.

Upon receiving her response, Śumbha arrogantly dispatched his general, Dhūmralocana, to drag her back to

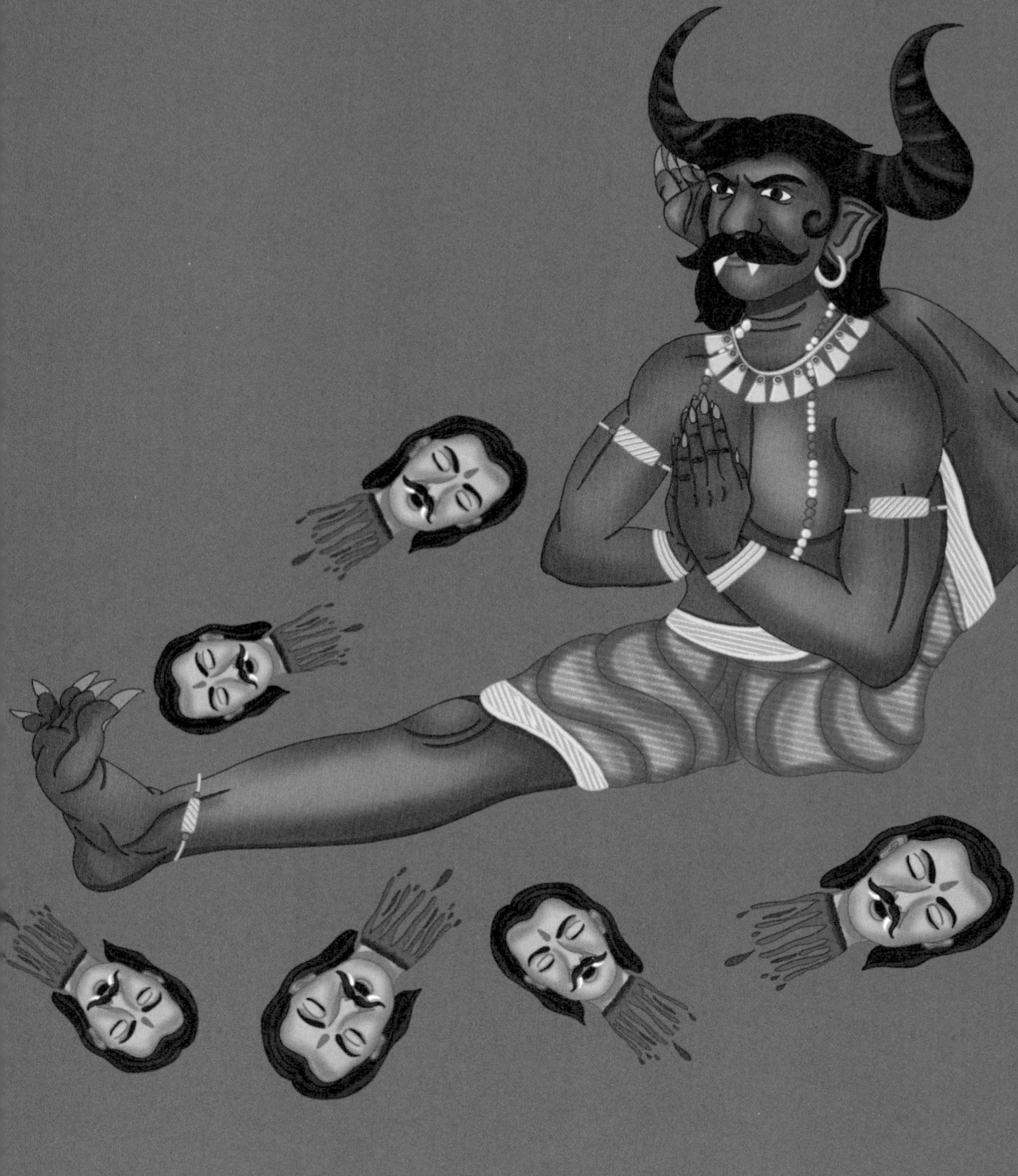

him by the hair. But, as Dhūmralocana approached, the goddess let out a single mantric utterance that reduced instantly him to ashes. Next, Śumbha decided to dispatch Caṇḍa and Muṇḍa, this time to bring the goddess to him against her will. As they made a dash for her, she scowled a terrible scowl and from between her knitted brow emerged a beam of light. From this beam coalesced the goddess Kālī, the terrible, with lolling tongue and garland of sculls, frightful to behold. Kālī decapitated Caṇḍa and Muṇḍa and brought their heads back to the goddess as a trophy. Having slain Caṇḍa and Muṇḍa, Kālī was given the name Cāmuṇḍa and praised by the gods for her heroism.

Śumbha couldn't take a hint from the incinerated Dhūmralocana or decapitated Caṇḍa and Muṇḍa, so he decided to release his secret weapon: the demon Raktabīja. Rāktabīja had a very special power: whenever a drop of his blood hit the earth, another Raktabīja was born. And to make matters worse, each Raktabīja clone had the same boon! Blind to the true nature of the feminine, Śumbha could not see the goddess as anything but an object of desire, and so, intent on possessing her, he marched his vast demonic hordes, including the menacing Raktabīja, into battle.

The goddess manifested an army of her own through her divine power. And from the bodies of the gods emerged goddesses to join the goddess' army. This army of special goddesses was called the Seven Mothers. From Brahmā's body emerged Brahmāṇi with prayer beads and water pot; from Śiva (Maheśvara) came Maheśvari astride a bull, trident in hand; from Kārttikeya (Kumāra), the god of war, sprang forth Kaumārī with readied spear; from Viṣṇu emerged Vaiṣṇavī, mounted on the eagle Garuḍa, with discus in hand; from Viṣṇu's bird incarnation came Vārāhī, and from his lion-man incarnation came Nārasiṃhī; from Indra emerged Aindrī, with lightning bolt in hand. The Seven Mothers and Kālī joined the army of the goddess and engaged Śumbha's demonic forces in a great battle.

The battle waged on between the goddess' forces and Śumbha's, arrows flying, swords clashing, spears piercing, axes hacking. The army of the goddess was winning, until Śumbha unleashed the terrible Raktabīja. Each blow that they dealt him only multiplied his presence upon the field of battle, and their own fierce prowess was turned against them. So, the goddess sent forth Kālī, to use her lolling tongue, and lap up every drop of blood before it hit the earth. In a maniacal frenzy, the mighty Kālī did just this, lapping up every single drop of blood in a gruesome manner. So it was that the goddess and her forces destroyed the demon army, Raktabījas and all. Enraged at the destruction of their army, Śumbha's brother Niśumbha made a mad dash to engage the goddess in one-on-one combat. Though he fought valiantly, he, too, perished at the hands of the mighty mother of the universe.

Śumbha, infuriated, his army destroyed, his brother slain, approached the goddess and addressed her thus: "You pathetic woman! You think you're so powerful, but all you ever do is rely on the strength of others. You would be nothing without Kālī, the Seven Mothers, and your army!"

The goddess replied, "It is you who rely on the strength of others, fool. These forces are nothing more than manifestations of my own power. I alone exist in all the worlds!" With that, she withdrew the forces into herself. Śumbha watched in terror, as Kālī, the Mothers, and the goddess' entire army were folded back into her very body. A great duel then waged between Śumbha and the goddess. The earth trembled and the oceans stirred as the two engaged in their cosmic duel. Finally, the goddess succeeded in decapitating the vile Śumbha. The earth calmed, the oceans receded, the dark clouds parted, and the sun shone down to signal the restoration of order caused by the goddess' triumph. The gods cheered at the victory of the goddess over their evil enemy! Their power was restored at long last, and the cosmic cycles returned to normal. Overjoyed, they raised their voices in glorious praise of the Mother Divine. Pleased by this, she granted them another boon, to which they asked that she quell all miseries for gods and mortals alike when called upon. The goddess pledged to return whenever needed, and promised that whomever will remember her deeds and chant her hymns will receive her blessings.

Decapitation as an instrument of divine grace is a recurring motif in Indic mythology, as well as in the story of the great goddess. The head represents the ego and the desires born of it. One can think of virtue as an awareness of everyone's ego, while vice is to have awareness of only one's own. The demons refused to give up their desires or destructive paths, so they needed to be decapitated to be stopped. When we are knocked off of a self-destructive or adharmic path, we are called to detach ourselves from egoic desires, just as the heads of so many arrogant figures are detached from their bodies in these tales. Those committed to the path of yoga do not need to be forcibly decapitated, because they voluntarily surrender their heads as an offering to the goddess. Just as bowing one's head connects one to the heart and quiets ego consciousness, so too does this pose occasion a surrender of self.

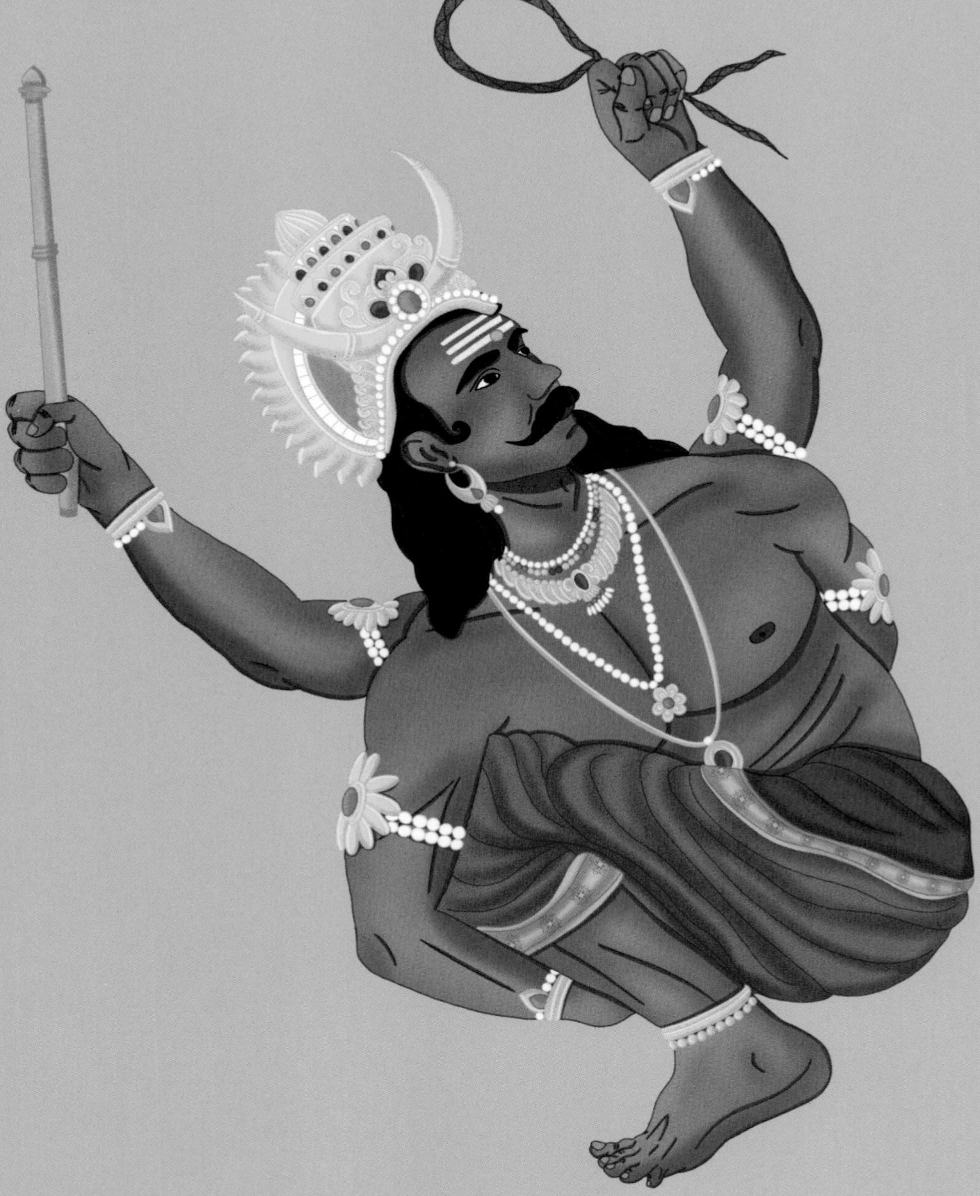

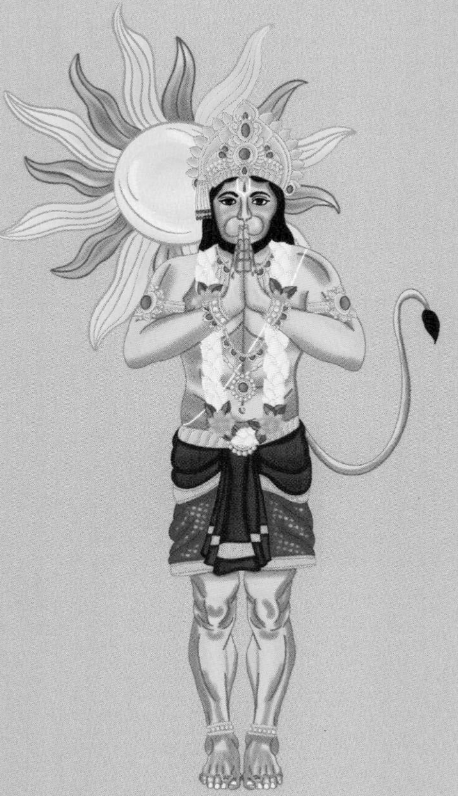

CHAPTER 4

The Power of the Gods

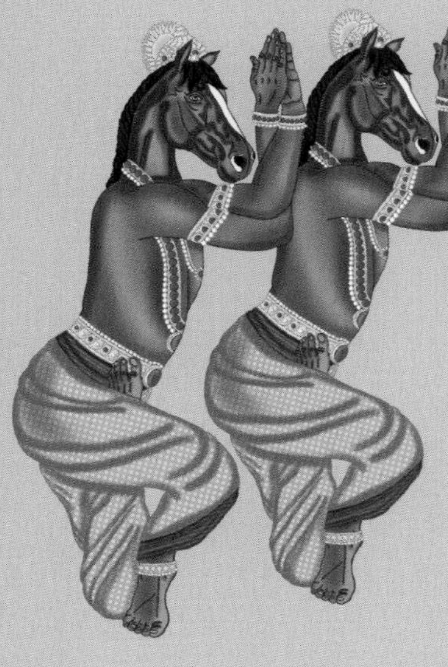

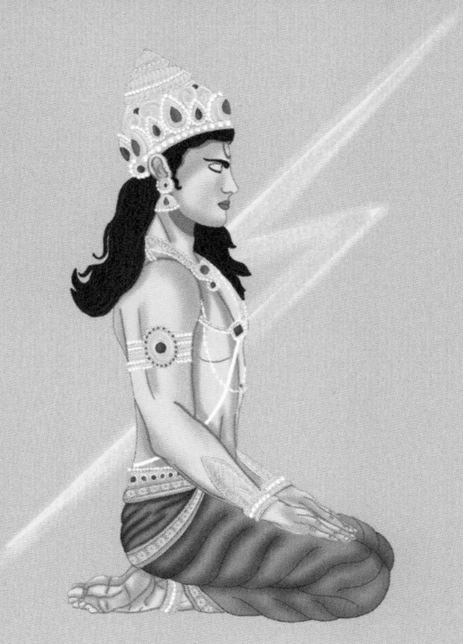

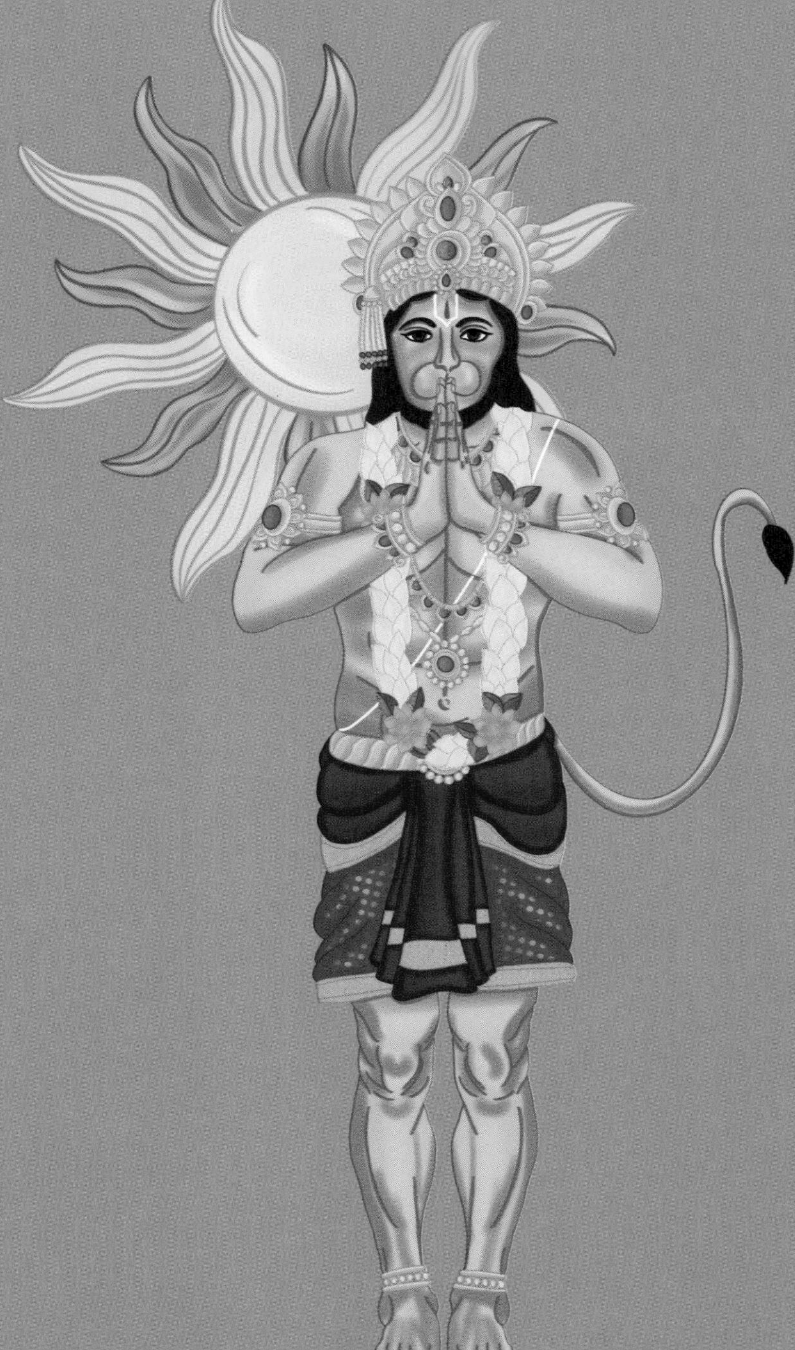

REVERENCE POSE
PRAṆĀMĀSANA

SALUTATIONS TO THE SUN

THEMES
Reverence
Centeredness
Inwardness

Hanumān was a very special monkey indeed, conceived by means of a special blessing from Lord Śiva himself. His mother, Añjanā, and father, Kesarī, were childless for some time, before Añjanā undertook penance to Śiva in order to obtain a son. She had long been a devotee of the Blue-Throated Lord, chanting his mantras and meditating on his form for decades with a sincere heart. So, Śiva decided to bless her with a very special son.

Śiva's seed was carried by the wind god, Vāyu, to Añjanā and with it, she conceived the great monkey hero Hanumān. From a very young age, he showed staggering feats of strength. As a young child, he could lift up his parents, and his spectacular strength only grew as he did. One morning, the young Hanumān was hungry, and his mother Añjanā was out at the market, buying mangoes, his favorite of all fruit. He looked out of his window and saw the rising sun, and mistook it for a ripe mango. So, with a push of his feet, he reached for the sun, and before he knew it, he was airborne! Hanumān travelled through the heavens, intent on reaching the sun. But just as he was nearing it, Indra, the king of heaven, intervened, saying, "This is no mango, child, this is the sun himself, bringer of day! You cannot go further, lest you perish by his flames!" With this, the disappointed Hanumān returned to earth. By this time, Añjanā returned from the market with a fresh basket of mangoes to sate her son's hunger. Though Hanumān ate his fill, he still thirsted for knowledge about the sun who he had come so close to meeting.

As Hanumān grew, he proved himself not only to be physically powerful, but also spiritually advanced. He was remarkably self-controlled, contained, content. He was happy to serve and he loved learning. While curiosity is natural for monkeys, his was of a different order. He was curious about how the world worked and the mysteries of life. He would seek out sages at every turn, to learn about virtue, wisdom, and truth. There came a time when he had learned all that he could from the elders of his clan, and still he wanted more. His childhood visit to the sun always stayed with him, but he now understood that his hunger for a juicy mango was actually a thirst for knowledge. So, the grown Hanumān set out toward the sun in search of truth.

Soaring through the heavens, Hanumān steered himself toward the sun. He soon drew near to the maker of day, effulgent, majestic, intense to behold. Sūrya, the sun god, was riding his chariot, drawn by seven celestial horses. Hanumān approached him and asked him for instruction. Sūrya refused on the basis that he was busy all day riding his chariot through the sky, and couldn't possibly stop to teach Hanumān. The clever monkey came up with a solution: "Glorious Sūrya, what if I keep pace with you, so that you may teach me all the while? Will you accept me as a student then?" Sūrya scoffed and said to Hanumān, "You can try if you'd like, but the longer you keep pace, the more exposure you'll have to my fiery presence. You'll be singed in no time!" Hanumān responded, "If you'll have me as a student, I'll keep pace for as long as I can. Even a day of your instruction is worth more than a lifetime without it." Sūrya agreed to instruct Hanumān.

Hanumān positioned himself to face the sun and flew backwards, matching the pace of his celestial chariot. And so Sūrya's instruction began. Sūrya taught him about Vedic knowledge and the mysteries of life. After all, the sun sees all, supports all, outlives all. He is the great bringer of illumination, possessing his own luster. The sun sees through shadows and can separate the wheat from the chaff. Hanumān learned a great deal, keeping pace with Sūrya day after day, week after week, month after month. Sūrya, impressed at the monkey's forbearance, intelligence, and respect, marched on with his teachings for exactly one year. When they were done, the wise and blackened Hanumān offered his prostrations to Sūrya, lord of day.

At the end of their training Sūrya asked Hanumān for a fee of his own choosing, knowing the monkey to be both considerate and wise. Hanuman replied: "Having learned from you the mysteries of being,

I wish not only to honor you as my guru for the rest of my days, but I want for all the world to honor you too. I know you are worshipped around the world with prayers and hymns, but I will devise a sequence of yoga postures dedicated to you. These postures will not only activate your solar energy within bodies of all who undertake them, but the sequence will also call them to reverence before your glory. The very first of these will be Praṇāmāsana, the position I adopt now as I pay my respects to you, guru sun."

Sūrya was pleased at this great gift, made in exchange for his yearlong instruction. He blessed Hanumān with success with his solar yoga sequence known to us as Sūrya Namaskāra.

Praṇāmāsana is the first step of Sūrya Namaskāra. It requires one to be centered, focused, and reverent. Whomever and whatever form our guru takes, we are called to respect them if we are to succeed in receiving all that they have to give. This posture naturally brings our attention to the heart center, so crucial for the mutual devotion flowing between teacher and student. The Sūrya Namaskāra sequence also calls us to lower our heads, and subdue our egos so that there is space to receive the grace our guru will give. Sūrya Namaskāra is far more than a heating practice geared toward the cultivation of the solar channel. It is a sequence that balances both channels, when done well. The sun is the light of awareness, representative of the light of the soul.

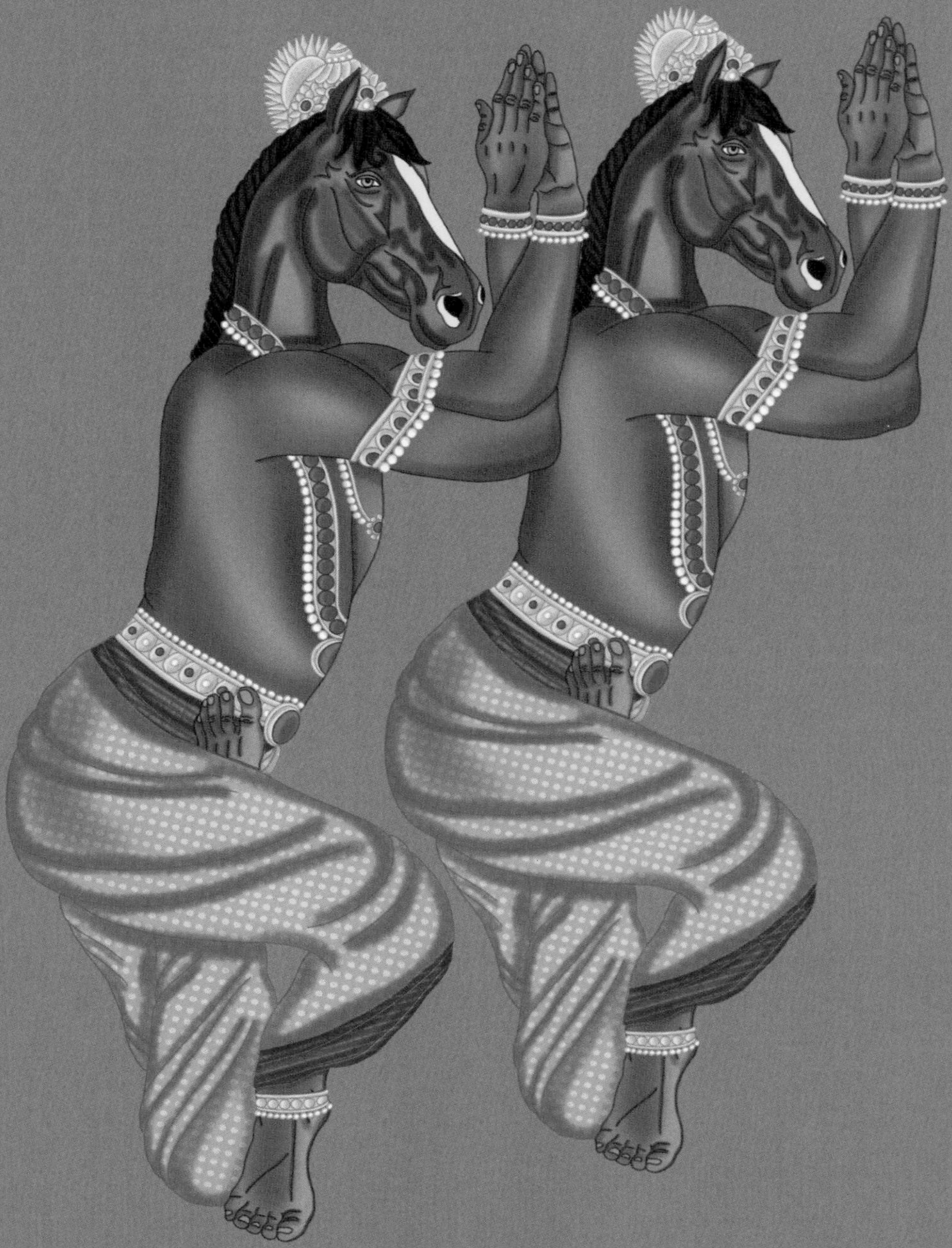

HORSE POSE
VĀTĀYANĀSANA

THE DIVINE HEALERS

THEMES
Patience
Persistence
Transformation

THE SUN AND HIS NEW WIFE SAṂJÑĀ lived happily at first. After all, they were very much in love, and Saṃjñā was swept off her feet, overjoyed to have Sūrya, the sun himself, as her own husband. They soon had three children, the eldest of which was Yama, the god of death. As time passed, the sun became more difficult to handle. He was glaring and overbearing, his heat unbearable. Saṃjñā couldn't take it anymore, so she created a duplicate of herself—Shadow—through the use of secret mantras. Saṃjñā instructed her Shadow, Chāyā, to stay in her stead, and to care for the sun and their 3 children. Chāyā agreed.

The sun, mistaking Chāyā for Saṃjñā, fathered another three children upon her. It soon became clear to Saṃjñā's eldest son, Yama, that Chāyā favored their younger three siblings for some reason. She scarcely paid any attention to Saṃjñā's children, and spent all her time and energy caring for her own. Yama decided to confront Chāyā, and was insolent toward her, threatening to kick her.

In response, she cursed Yama that his foot would fall off. Disturbed, Yama went to complain to Sūrya. Sūrya agreed that no matter how a son misbehaves, a mother would never curse him, and they both knew that something wasn't right. So, Sūrya confronted Chāyā about her ill treatment of their first three children, and she feigned ignorance. The sun then released his mighty glare, threatening to scorch Chāyā where she stood. She could not withstand him, and confessed the truth of the situation. Outraged, the sun went off in pursuit of Saṃjñā.

The sun went to his father-in-law Viśvakarman, the divine craftsman, to see if Saṃjñā was there. Viśvakarman mentioned that she had visited a while back, but had left, saying that she was returning home. The sun then looked inward with his yogic eye to see where Saṃjñā was. He spotted her, in the form of a mare, performing penance in the fields, hoping to find a solution to her unbearable situation. "I think I know what the issue is," said the sun to Viśvakarman. "My glare is too overbearing. Since you are creation's greatest craftsman, tinkerer bar none, the divine architect himself, would you please use your divine tools to temper my radiance, so that my beloved Saṃjñā may bear my presence?" Viśvakarman agreed and went to work chipping away at the luster of the sun until he was bearable to the naked eye. Sūrya then assumed equine form himself and galloped toward his beloved Saṃjñā. The two, delighted to see each other, conceived right then and there. So came into being the Aśvin twins, the horse-headed divine healers of the gods. Seeing that her husband had tempered his glare, Saṃjñā gladly returned home, enjoying his benign form.

The Aśvin twins are an ever-youthful, strong, and handsome pair. They are brilliant, golden in hue like their father, and swift like the wind. They are also compassionate, always willing to help cure diseases, and ride in the sun's chariot each morning to help create the day. Once, they were called on to help heal sage Cyavana, who was quite aged at the time. The sage's wife Sukanyā said to them: "Though you share in the beauty and the skill of the gods, I know you do not share in their immortality. I of course cannot grant you immortality myself, but I know what you must do to attain it. If you can heal my husband, I will share what I know." The twins, already called by their love of healing, were now especially motivated to cure Cyavana. So, they anointed him with special herbs into which they incanted secret mantras. Then, they led him to a holy pond, and instructed him to immerse himself in it. Cyavana emerged reborn from the holy waters in a youthful, healthy state. Overjoyed at her husband's good health, Sukanyā made good on her promise: "In order to attain immortality, noble Aśvins, you must imbibe *soma*, the elixir of life. And in order to do so, you must find a sage who knows how to prepare the sacrifice. I know such a sage, his name is Dadhīchi. Go to him and he will help."

The Aśvins tracked down Dadhīchi, and he was indeed happy to oblige. "I will gladly perform the ritual for you," said Dadhīchi. "But there's one problem. Indra, king of heaven, guards the elixir, and he has issued the curse that the head of anyone who performs the ritual will burst into a thousand pieces! So, if you can somehow find a way to thwart Indra, then the soma sacrifice shall be yours." The Aśvins came up with an ingenious plan that only they, with their knowledge of anatomy and gifts for healing, could accomplish. They replaced the sage's head with that of a horse, keeping the sage's head alive and well. Once Dadhīchi performed the ritual granting immortality to the Aśvins, his horse head burst into a thousand pieces. The Aśvins then successfully reattached his real head, successfully safeguarding Dadhīchi from Indra's curse.

Horses are symbols of strength and vitality, associated with health and healing in the Indian context. They are also connected with the sun, another symbol of wellness and vitality. While cows embody the feminine principle, horses embody masculinity, vitality, and virility. Nevertheless, Sūrya's overbearing masculinity needs to be tempered by the feminine and brought into balance. He therefore submits to Saṃjñā's father, the divine architect, to be hammered down for the sake of his relationship with Saṃjñā. Having attained a balanced state, the sun fathers the equine divine healers, the Aśvin twins. Unlike Sūrya, the twins are mild, modest, and always a pleasure to behold. Their own quest for immortality is brought to fruition by a sage with a horse's head, again, signalling the significance of equine energy for all matters of health, longevity, and even immortality. Meditate on the twists and turns of the tale of the Aśvins as you undertake this difficult pose. One foot is firmly planted, and you have the head of a horse, but the other foot is in half lotus, invoking the sage who performs the sacred soma sacrifice. This pose is a challenging one, requiring you to adopt the patience, persistence, and ingenuity found in the divine healer.

HALF-MOON POSE

ARDHACANDRĀSANA

BALANCING HEAVEN AND EARTH

THEMES
Balance
Awareness
Grounding

THE MOON GOD (CANDRA) was handsome, charming, debonair. He was full of light and a joy to be around. His mild, benign temperament was enjoyed by all, and he certainly knew how to have fun! He would gallivant around the heavens in his antelope-drawn chariot. A creature of whim, Candra fluttered from interest to interest like the social butterfly he was. But to whomever his attention was focused upon, he was deeply empathetic, a good listener, and a comfort. He also had a wild imagination, and a profound intuition. But commitment wasn't among his virtues.

When time came to get married, Candra found an arrangement that was suitable to his temperament. It just so happened that at that time, Dakṣa, son of Brahmā, was looking for grooms for his 27 daughters. When Candra came to meet the potential brides, he was quite taken with every one of them, able to empathize and connect with each. And all of Dakṣa's daughters were dazzled by his charming presence. They all asked Dakṣa if they could be his bride. With all of his daughters more than willing, Dakṣa was at a loss for how to proceed, so he asked Candra to name the bride of his choice. Candra said he would like to marry all of them! The brides-to-be were absolutely delighted, and so the marriage was arranged. Mesmerized by the moon, each bride agreed to be with him once every 27 nights, so all of

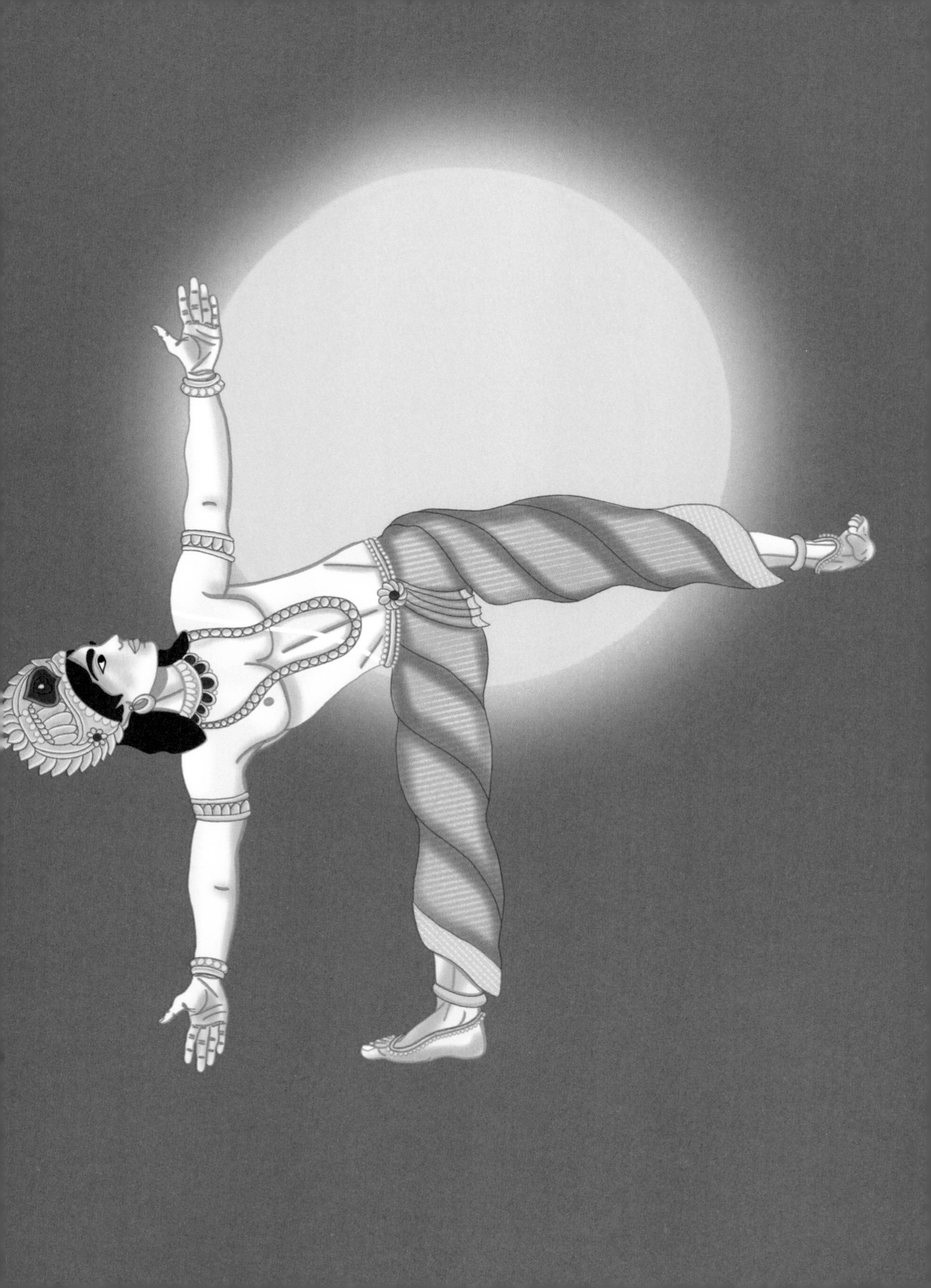

them could have a turn. Flamboyant romantic that he was, Candra was ecstatic at the arrangement and looked forward to connecting with each of his brides.

Dakṣa's daughter Rohini was the youngest and fairest of them all, and the moon secretly desired her more intensely than the others. When it came her turn to spend the night with the moon god, they became deeply engrossed in each other, savoring every moment of their passion and tenderness. When the next day came, the moon could not pull himself away from Rohini, and so, he stayed with her for a second night, and then a third, and this went on for weeks! Finally, after 26 nights had passed, all of the 26 remaining neglected daughters of Dakṣa went to complain to their father. They expressed their outrage at being neglected as young newlyweds. And, of course, they were naturally jealous of the attention that Rohini was getting. So, they insisted Dakṣa do something.

Dakṣa decided to intervene in his daughters' unjust treatment. He set out to Candra's abode immediately and confronted him about his outrageous behavior:

"Father Dakṣa, what's the problem?" Candra responded. "I'm enjoying myself with Rohini, and she's definitely enjoyed herself with me!"

"Be that as it may, Candra, life is not all about enjoyments! You have a responsibility to be there for all of your wives."

"Surely they knew what they were getting into when they married me, Father Dakṣa? It was my free-spirited indulgence that endeared me to them in the first place."

Furious, Dakṣa replied, "Since you are so satisfied with your own luster, the very same that blinds you to decency, I curse you to lose your shine! We'll see how enjoyable life is for you then."

With that, Dakṣa immediately departed back to his abode, and the moon started to lose his luster. He was beside himself, wallowing in grief and self-pity. He pined away, day after day, losing a sliver each night until, after a fortnight, he had lost his lustre entirely. This dark night of the soul was painful and disorienting for him indeed. What is a peacock without its tail? Painful as this ordeal was, it was also instructive. It taught him humility and respect, and how to act out of responsibility instead of desire. He spent a night with each wife as was his husbandly duty. But both he and his wives really missed his luster, and the heavens were not quite the same without it. So, Candra took up penance to Lord Śiva. After some time, Lord Śiva, pleased, appeared before him. He asked the lord to reverse Dakṣa's curse, to which Śiva replied,"My dear Candra, I cannot reverse Dakṣa's curse, but I can modify it. Since you are truly repentant and changed by your loss of lustre, I want to leave you without it. But since many of your qualities shine forth through your luster, I want to grant that to you as well."

"Lord Śiva, I do not understand. Will I be bright or dark?"

"Both," replied Lord Śiva with a twinkle in his eye. "All things oscillate through the sway of time, and hence forth, so too will you. For a fortnight you will wax in luster until Dakṣa's curse is eclipsed by your brightness, then, at the very moment you attain your full luster, you will start to lose it again over the course of a second fortnight, and this will appease Dakṣa's curse. It shall be so until I dance destruction upon the universe at the end of time." Candra bowed deeply before the lord, grateful for his blessing. And to this day, the moon waxes and wanes across the heavens.

The waxing moon is associated with outwardness, social connection, and indulging pleasures, while the waning moon is associated with inwardness, isolation, and sense-withdrawal. The new moon can be understood as when our awareness is completely internalized, perhaps in meditative posture. It was in this state that the moon was able to commune with Śiva. When we are able to let go of our ego and sense-gratification, we are able to diligently perform our duties and serve others. And yet there's more to life than self-abnegation. The full moon represents joviality and festivity. This is the energy of social gatherings, connections, pleasure, and general joie de vivre. And so, the human experience needs to oscillate between the two to find balance. The exact midpoint is the half-moon, after which this posture is named. Reflect on the story of the moon when engaging this posture, for the key to it is finding your balance between heaven and earth, between supine and upstanding postures.

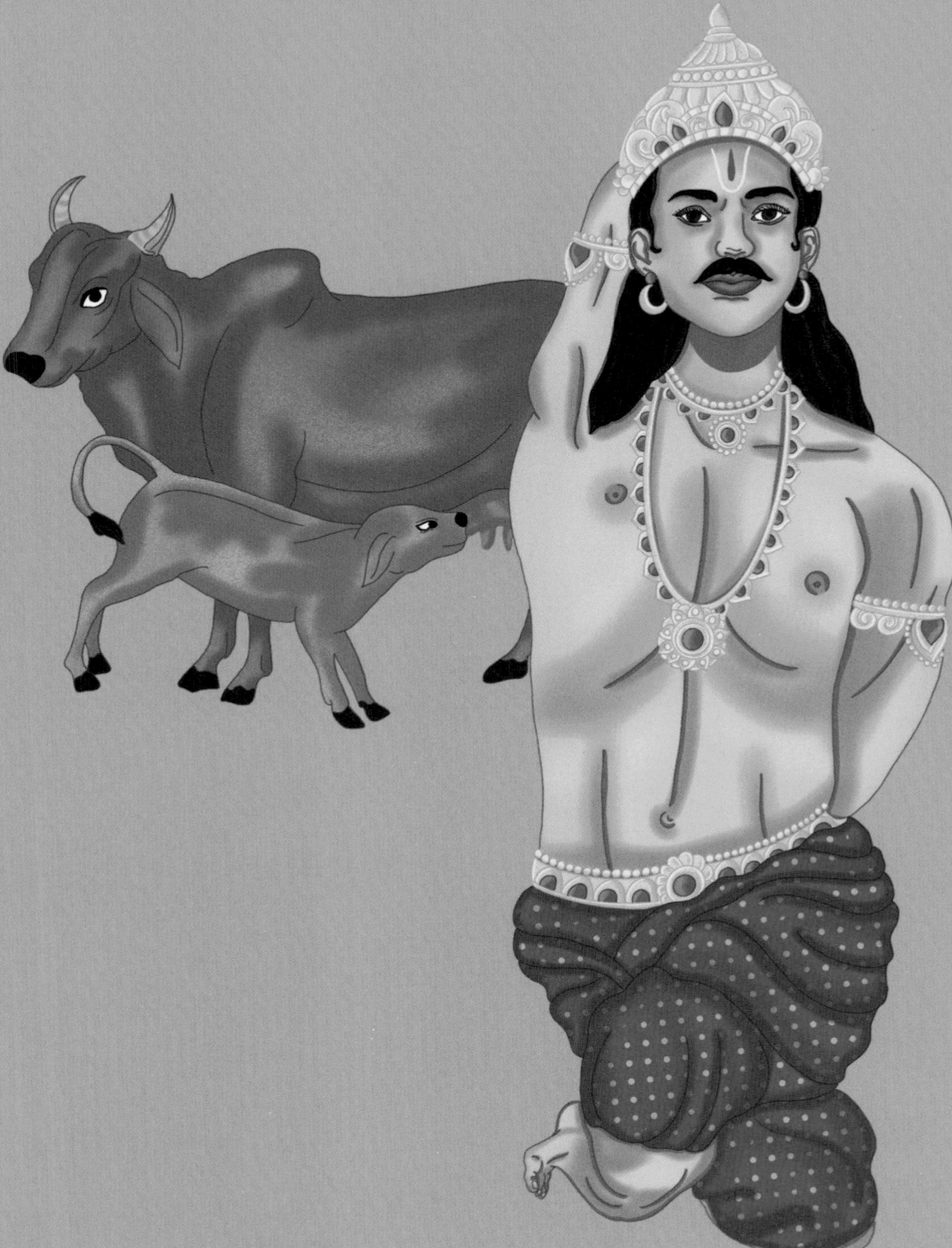

COW FACE POSE
GOMUKHĀSANA

DIVINE
NURTURANCE

THEMES
Stretching
Softness
Grounding

THERE ONCE WAS A MAN NAMED VENA who was so power-hungry, that he conquered all the lands he could, and declared himself sovereign over the world. He was a self-serving tyrant, the sort of person least suited for power. And yet, it is just such folks who end up scrambling for such positions. He taxed the citizens mercilessly, and raped and pillaged the earth for his own gain. He was constantly digging for silver, gold, and precious gems. He did as he pleased without regard for the welfare of his citizens. He became so conceited that one day, he called all of the sages into his court and decreed that they were no longer to perform Vedic sacrifices. He informed them that since he was richer and greater than the gods of heaven, it was he who should be worshipped. The sages tried to reason with him, explaining that their rituals upheld the very rhythms of the cosmos and without them, calamity would ensue. King Vena didn't care about any of that, as long as he had the riches, position, and attention he needed to satisfy his ego. And so, under fear of death, the sages immediately discontinued their sacred rituals.

With the ceasing of the sacred rituals, the atmosphere changed around the world. The lands heated up, and the rains stopped falling. Mother Earth, already depleted thanks to King Vena's greedy excavations, suffered still more greatly from the cessation of the rains. At her wit's end, and exhausted by Vena's abuse, she turned herself into a cow and ran away to protect herself from the madness. When Mother Earth withdrew her energy from the planet, the crops withered and lakes and rivers dried up. Calamity loomed across the land; citizens starved and nature was thrown into imbalance. But King Vena didn't care. All he cared about was himself and the power he wielded over others. He had already amassed a storehouse of grain that would last for years, so he was content to sit back and let the earth perish, and his citizens with it.

The court sages were livid. They could not sit around and allow the word to crumble. They needed to remove King Vena, but they had a problem. Force was the duty of kings, whose function it was to protect the sages. But in the absence of such protection, the sages had to protect themselves and the realm. So, they plucked a blade of kuśa grass from the withering fields and consecrated it with special mantras. The blade of grass was plunged into King Vena's heart, and he was finally dethroned. But now, the sages had another problem: who would replace him? Vena had no heir. So, they performed a ritual using Vena's corpse, churning it to procure an heir. At first their churning yielded a wicked dwarf, which was the crystallization of Vena's vice. Then, after some time, a handsome, noble, kingly figure emerged. They named him Pṛthu and installed him as the very first consecrated Indian king.

King Pṛthu well understood that the primary dharma of the king is to protect—to protect citizens, sages, even the earth itself, whenever the need arises. His first order as king was to have the sages immediately resume the sacred rituals. He needed all the blessings he could get, given the dire calamity he had inherited. His citizens were starving, and Mother Earth had withdrawn her energy from the planet. It was by the divine sight of one of the sages that Pṛthu came to know that Mother Earth had taken the form of a cow, to gallop far away from Vena and his treachery. So, Pṛthu mounted his horse and set out to find her.

King Pṛthu searched far and wide without rest until he spotted the divine embodiment of the fecundity of Earth itself. As he approached her, she trotted away more quickly for fear of being abused further. The king cut her off at a pass and spoke these words:

"Great Mother, fear not! I am not the vile Vena; I am his successor Pṛthu. I come in peace and respect, to beseech you to please return and rejuvenate the earth. My people are dying without your grace."

"Lord Pṛthu, I can do no such thing. For which sensible, self-respecting sentient being would allow themselves to be abused? I can be raped and pillaged no more, and so I must flee."

"Mother, hear me out," Pṛthu pleaded. "I ache, knowing of your abuse at the greedy hands of King Vena. I do not approach you for riches or gold, only food for my starving people. It is not in the spirit of greed I address you, but in the spirit of need. You have my solemn word that as king, I will protect you, and ensure that my citizens reap from your bounty in a reasonable manner. And so it will be for all of my successors."

Seeing the sincerity in King Pṛthu's eyes, the divine cow spoke these words: "A mother's duty is to unconditionally love, accept, and nurture all of her children, and so I have, for countless millennia. A mother's duty is not to accept abuse from anyone, least of all her own children. Moved by your words, and trusting your promise, I will submit to you to be milked so that the earth may be replenished. But though cows may consent to give milk, they must be fed and honored in return. I accept you as my protector, and from this day forth I will be known as Pṛthvī, the ward of Pṛthu and his heirs. But remember this: should you ever abuse me again, the people of earth shall suffer from fire, floods, and disease."

Pṛthu was overjoyed at Mother Earth's return, as were the people of Earth. He protected the welfare of the Earth for the rest of his days and ensured that he passed down Pṛthvī's pledge to his heirs.

The cow is greatly revered in the Indian context. It is a gentle, calm, kind animal who selflessly serves at every turn. From the cow is gotten milk, butter, and ghee. The cow is a ready symbol for the sacred feminine and its capacity to nurture. Hence the cow makes the perfect personification—and analogue—of the Earth's capacity to nurture. In short, both cow and Earth exemplify motherhood. The sacred feminine is to be cherished and protected. Viṣṇu the Preserver is sworn to protect the universe, battling demons at every turn, even personally incarnating to do so. One of his most famous incarnations was that of Kṛṣṇa, who, interestingly was raised as a cowherder, sworn to protect cows. As you engage this pose, call to mind the affable, benign generous nature of cows. Reflect also on the cow as exemplar of the all-nurturing sacred feminine, an analogue to the earth itself.

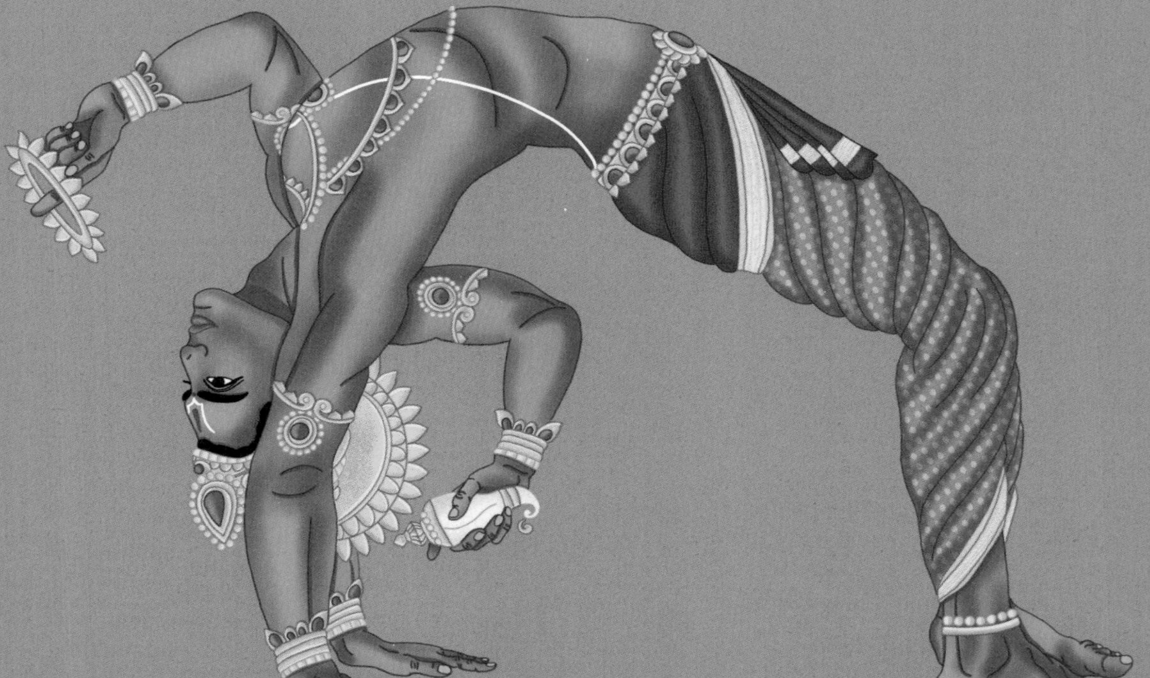

WHEEL POSE
CAKRĀSANA

EMBODYING VIṢṆU'S DISCUS

THEMES
Light
Darkness
Awareness

LONG AGO, THE GODS AND DEMONS worked together to procure the Elixir of Immortality. In order to do so, they needed to churn the cosmic ocean, source of all things. Mount Meru was used as a churning pole, around which was wrapped Vāsuki, king of serpents, who volunteered his body to be used as a churning rope. Viṣṇu himself, the great Preserver, incarnated as a great sea tortoise and swam to the bottom of the ocean so that Mount Meru could be placed on his back. The gods lined up on one side, the demons on the other, and together, they began the arduous work of churning the oceans in search of the elixir. Soon after they began churning, a substance emerged from the oceans and shot straight up in the air. The demons and gods were delighted, thinking it was the elixir. But their delight soon turned to horror once they realized that the substance was poison! The great god Śiva, seeing with his third eye what was happening, came upon the scene in haste. He opened his mouth and allowed the poison to descend into it. If Śiva swallowed the poison, he would die, and if he spat it out, all assembled would perish instead. So, Śiva found a third option: he neutralized the poison in his throat, neither swallowing it nor spitting it out. His neck turned a deep shade of blue, and from that day forth, he was praised as the Blue-Throated Lord!

After Śiva was praised, the churning continued. For eons the churning went on, as various riches emerged from the cosmic oceans. Among them were Indra's five-headed elephant, Kāmadhenu the cow of plenty, the wish-fullfilling tree, various nymphs, precious gems, and even Lakṣmī, goddess of abundance, emerged from the cosmic churning. At long last, the sage Dhanvantarī, father of Ayurveda emerged, holding an effulgent pot. Instantly, the demons and gods knew what was inside—the elixir of life, at long last procured! The gods knew they needed the help of the demons to churn the celestial ocean, but they never intended to share it, since immortality should belong to the gods alone. The gods had always meant to steal the elixir away at the crucial moment, but, predictably enough, the demons had come up with the exact same plan! So, both factions made a mad dash for the ambrosial vessel, but the covetous demons got there first. The gods were horrified, having endured such great toil only to have given the demons the upper hand. Aghast, they called to Viṣṇu for help.

It was, of course, Viṣṇu's role to preserve order throughout the universe. So, he devised a plan to deal with the demons. He knew that neither reasoning nor bartering would work, so he adopted the only viable strategy that remained: trickery. He disguised himself in feminine form, donning the garb of the great nymph, Mohinī , an embodiment of infatuation itself. The demons' attentions were captured by Mohinī and so, distracted, they lost interest in the elixir, in pursuit of sensual pleasures. To this day Mohinī evades them, for she is nothing more than a projection of Viṣṇu, smoke and mirrors, deployed to distract them. Disaster averted, the gods secured the pot of ambrosia and carried it off to their heavenly abode.

Seated in a circle in their sacred assembly hall, the gods began their festivities as each god, in turn, imbibed a drop of the elixir and attained immortality. Although the demons were fooled by Viṣṇu's ruse, the greatest trickster among them, Rāhu, saw through it. He was himself a master of disguises, so when all of his demon comrades went off in pursuit of Mohinī , he disguised himself as one of the gods and snuck into the assembly hall to join the festivities. Seated in the sacred circle, Rāhu salivated as he awaited his taste of ambrosial bliss. Eventually it was Rāhu's turn to receive the vessel. He raised it above his head and tipped it such that a single drop of precious ambrosia fell toward his eager tongue. But Rāhu was seated between the gods of the sun and moon, and in that moment, illuminating the scene with their own light, they were able to see through the demon's disguise. The sun god exclaimed, "Viṣṇu, there is a demon among us!"

Viṣṇu jumped to his feet and launched his divine discus, the Sudarśana Cakra. It sailed through the air, toward the neck of the demon Rāhu, just as the drop of elixir simultaneously fell fatefully toward his tongue. If the elixir landed first, Rāhu would attain immortality and become impervious to the discus. But, if the discus arrived first, he would be dead and would not attain immortality. But the drop of elixir passed into his throat at the very moment the discuss decapitated him. The discus returned to Viṣṇu's hand, having done its deadly deed. The demon Rāhu was now two immortal demons: a body without a head (Ketu) and a head without a body (Rāhu). Rahu chases the sun and the moon to this day, having never forgiven them for blowing his cover. When he catches up, he swallows them, but having no body, they pass straight through him. The conjunction of Rahu and the sun marks a solar eclipse, and when Rahu gobbles up the moon, it creates a lunar eclipse. Such is the power of Viṣṇu's discus to decapitate demons in the blinking of an eye, swifter than the time it takes for a drop of elixir to reach your tongue.

Among the many foes that Viṣṇu's discus has decapitated, perhaps the most captivating story is that of the demon Rāhu. Much like the light of the sun and the moon, the discus destroys darkness, decapitating demons for the sake of heightened awareness. In wheel pose, your body adopts a circular form, while planting your hands and feet firmly on the ground. This posture represents the whirling of Viṣṇu's discuss, known as his "wheel", or "cakra". Pronounced "chakra" in Sanskrit, this is the same word used for the wheels of life located at our sacred centers (chakras).

ARCHER POSE
DHANURĀSANA

ARJUNA'S AIM

THEMES
Tension
Attention
Balance

Long ago, Earth stood upon the brink of a cataclysmic war between two great and powerful dynasties, the Pāṇḍavas (the children of Pāṇḍu) and the Kauravas (the descendants of Kuru). Both houses originated from the same lineage, but they had become estranged, and after many sleights and much political maneuvering, tensions had escalated, and all attempts at peaceful resolution had failed. Even Kṛṣṇa, an incarnate form of Viṣṇu himself, could not preserve the peace. The fate of humanity was at stake. War had become unavoidable.

The greatest warrior of the Pāṇḍavas was Arjuna. His skill with a bow was unparalleled, and he was the most beloved student of Droṇācārya, the great guru of military arts, who had trained him and his brothers since they were young boys. Arjuna and Kṛṣṇa were longstanding companions and great friends who had stuck together through thick and thin throughout many previous adventures. When both the Pāṇḍavas and Kauravas asked for the help of Kṛṣṇa and his army in their fight against one another, Kṛṣṇa determined that he himself would side with one of the great houses, but without entering personally into combat, while his army would fight for the other. He gave Arjuna first choice, who immediately chose that he would have his friend by his side, regardless of the consequences.

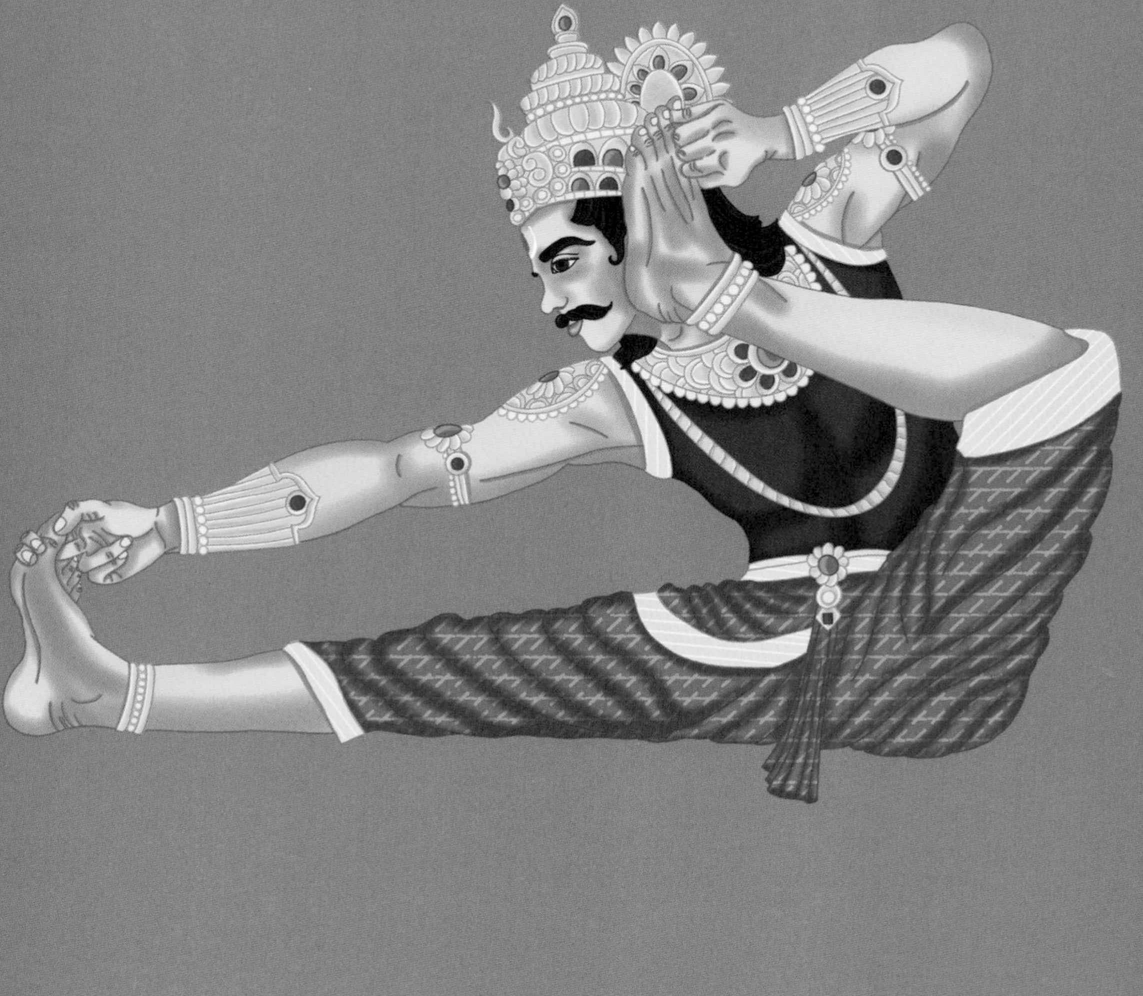

So it was, that at the fateful moment, just before the commencement of the great battle, Kṛṣṇa drove his famous chariot up to the front lines, escorting his beloved companion, the great archer, into the center of the scene. But as they came upon a place where Arjuna could first see the enemy, a heavy burden of sadness spread through him. The so-called enemy was composed of men he knew; cousins and uncles, acquaintances, and friends stood before him. He became heavy as lead, and lay down in the chariot, stricken as though himself hit with an arrow to the heart.

"Kṛṣṇa, I cannot do this dreadful thing, slaughtering my kith and kin. I see now the wisdom of the ascetics, and will take up a begging bowl and renounce the world. The wise say this is the way of virtue."

But Kṛṣṇa had made his peace with the necessity of the war. He saw the greater forces at play, and though his compassion was incomparable in scope, he chastised Arjuna in this moment, compelling him to stand up and regain his fighting spirit.

"You certainly parrot wise words, Arjuna, but you are not wise, for where there is true wisdom, there is no grief, neither for the living nor the dead. Where light shines forth, there can be no darkness. We are all eternal, Arjuna, be not fooled by these roles we play from life to life."

Arjuna was still paralyzed by confusion and doubt. Here was the Great Preserver himself, instructing him to let loose his murderous abilities upon his own people, contradicting all the fibers of his being, which told him to lay down his arms and seek a life of peace. But his faith in Kṛṣṇa was unwavering, and he knew that he must trust in his wisdom, so he asked question after question, and though the grief refused to leave him, he listened as Kṛṣṇa patiently answered every inquiry. Kṛṣṇa reminded him of the impermanence of all created beings, and the divine continuity that lay behind and beyond the mundane world:

"Never was there a time when I did not exist, nor you, nor anyone who stands about us on this field of battle; nor in the future shall any of us cease to exist."

He told Arjuna that there was no sense in trying to fight against the role that had been handed to him to carry out; that it is better to strive to carry out one's role with devotion and clarity than it is to pine after a different part in the divine play:

"You are a warrior; your duty is as such. To be in accordance with your dharma, you must pick up your bow and let your arrows fly. If, however, you choose to resist your religious duty, only then will you have been neglectful. Concern yourself not with the outcomes of your actions, and think only to carry them out well, as your duty demands.

You are not the cause of the consequences, to think such is mere attachment."

And, again and again, Kṛṣṇa warned Arjuna not to put too much stock in this temporary world of finite lifespans and decaying illusion, and to instead focus on the bigger picture: on the eternal, the absolute; the infinite and timeless divinity that lay behind all things.

"Now, gentle Arjuna," said Kṛṣṇa, "how well have you been listening? Well enough, I hope, that your ignorance and illusion are now dispelled?"

At this moment, strength returned to Arjuna, and he stood, once again, erect in his chariot. He clutched his great Gāṇḍīva bow and declared to Kṛṣṇa, "By your infinite grace, my doubts are gone. I am ready to fight!"

The exchange between Kṛṣṇa and Arjuna is a powerful metaphor for the battle between good and evil within one's psyche. It also offers us a way to engage the world, without becoming overly enmeshed in it. Kṛṣṇa's counsel to Arjuna is to embrace the ascetic ideologies of ancient India without eschewing the world, and falling prey to escapism. We have a duty to the world, as well as one toward enlightenment. And both duties are to be carried out in tandem, engaging the world while remaining unattached; cultivating compassion, but also, wisdom. In this great battle of life, we all need to stand tall. Your gaze should find the horizon, where heaven and earth meet. The horizon is the space of human experience, wherein Kṛsṇa's practical spiritual counsel applies. We need to go forth and do our duty, for others depend upon it. Everybody has a part to play—the world itself depends upon the balance of karma and dharma.

Arjuna's arrow represents his power to aim and meet his target. To meet our own goals, we also require a combination of vision, action, and strength. The flight of the arrow is dependent not only upon the archer's aim, but also upon the constitution of the bow. Without adequate tension in the string, the arrow will not fly. But with too much, the bow might break. In life, we must strive for a similar balance, being wound tightly enough that we can generate the vitality we need to move through the world, but not so tightly that we snap or burn out. In arrow pose, the same principles apply. Know the limits of your body, and engage and apply tension accordingly. Feel into this posture and become attuned to yourself. Balancing tension and strength is the foundation of good aim.

TREE POSE
VṚKṢĀSANA

STRETCHED BETWEEN HEAVEN AND EARTH

THEMES
Connection
Stability
Growth

Once, the great Sage Mārkaṇḍeya had been in deep meditation for eons on end when a great storm swept the earth. The deluge marked the end of the age; the destruction of all things was upon him. The waters would soon envelop the earth in preparation for cosmic dissolution. Having just come out of his meditation, Mārkaṇḍeya wasn't at all frightened. He was centered and ready to embrace what came. He simply marvelled at the great torrents of rain being pelted down from the perturbed heavens. Soon, a wave swept him up in its whirling fury and carried him off. As far as the eye could see, water covered the earth. He was carried by the currents to the top of a massive wave, where, held mysteriously in place, was a great banyan tree. "This could be no ordinary banyan," thought Mārkaṇḍeya, "for it is not rooted in soil, but in water, in the middle of this great expanse. How could it possibly survive here? And yet it thrives!" The mysterious banyan tree in the middle of the ocean was glowing with great splendor, a sight to behold. To Mārkaṇḍeya's great delight, the current that carried him delivered him to its base. Mesmerized, he approached the tree and noticed that upon one of its branches sat a smiling child.

Mārkaṇḍeya approached the radiant child in awe, wondering if this was a dream, or vision. He reached to pick

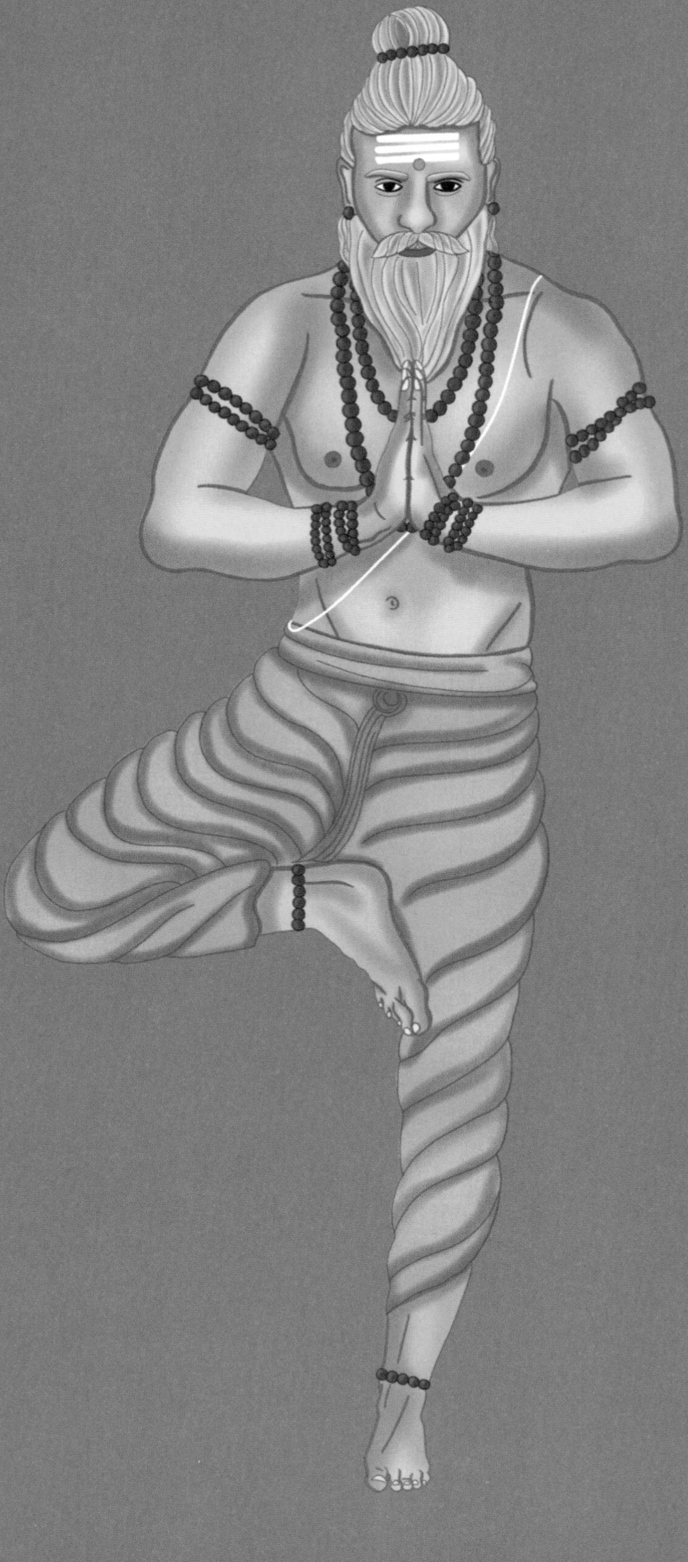

up the child, but just as he did so, the child took a deep breath in. Now, Mārkaṇḍeya found himself swept up again, as though by another great wave, but this time he was carried on the currents of the air being sucked into the child's mouth! Either the child's mouth grew in size, or Mārkaṇḍeya had shrunk—he couldn't tell—because before he knew it, he was able to comfortably enter the mouth of the child, as if it were the mouth of some mystical cave where great masters go to become enlightened. Once inside the mouth of this strange child, Mārkaṇḍeya beheld the entire surface of the earth, as it was before the flood. He beheld the jungles, the mountains, and the plains. He cast his gaze upwards and was inebriated at the expanse of the sky before him. He was somehow able to see the sun in its full glory, the brimming moon, and the vast array of stars lighting up the night sky. Further yet, his gaze met the galactic expanse, and the planets, stars, and galaxies making up the universe—and all in the mouth of the child! Mārkaṇḍeya soon realized that he must be standing in the mouth of the great god Viṣṇu, who pervades the world and envelops it at the end of the age.

The cosmic child then exhaled, and just as Mārkaṇḍeya had been drawn rapidly into the body of the child, so, too, was he thrust back out of his mouth, back into the presence of the majestic banyan. Mārkaṇḍeya sat at the base of the tree, taking solace from the great banyan, even in the midst of the great deluge. He meditated upon the presence of the tree that held within its boughs the divine presence.

Trees are peaceful, silent, still, present, and therefore make suitable sites not only for yogic practice, but also for yogic perfection. Many a sage has attained enlightenment beneath a tree, perhaps most famously, the Indian Prince Siddhartha Gautama who renounced and found enlightenment beneath the bodhi tree. The tree is both symbol and exemplar of profound wisdom. Humans can learn much from their majesty. For humans to be fullfilled, they need to continually grow, as trees do. The tree is taller each day than the day before. It stretches outwards and upwards toward the expanse of the sky. The sky is the space of ideas, ideals, and truths. It is the plane of the heavens, of divinity, of the beyond. And the tree is wise to stretch itself, becoming more than it was before, in an effort to touch the sky. We are wise to follow suit. In addition to being a plane of magic and wonder, the sky is home to the sun, source of heat and light. The sun represents the self within all beings, that spiritual spark of awareness, animation, grace which propels all life. As the tree ceaselessly receives the sun's grace, so too should we. In our goings and comings upon the earth, do we take the time to gaze upon the sky? Do you make space for wonder when you behold the sun, moon, and stars? Trees know well the wisdom of communing with the sky, yet they do not operate with their head in the clouds.

The secret to the tree's growth lies in its opposed impulses. Its impulse to reach up, into the sky is matched and made possible by its capacity to burrow down, deep into the earth. The tree's growth is literally dependent upon its groundedness, and this holds within it great wisdom. The tree gains support and stability by digging deep, its roots reaching toward the centre of the earth. The tree is testament to the fecundity of the earth, whereby it grows. It digs deep into the cool, moist earth to derive hydration and nourishment. It is not only fed by the earth, but also nourishes the earth with its fallen leaves and fruit. The symbolism of the tree calls us toward symbiotic participation in Earth's grand network of life. The tree's downward pull toward the earth represents its feminine aspect. While its upward pull toward the sky represents its masculine aspect. The power of the tree lies in its ability to integrate masculine and feminine: its upward growth is dependent upon its downward growth, and its downward growth eis equally dependent upon its upwards growth. The tree is whole, complete, and at peace.

Tree pose is, to some, a simple pose, but for those who know the great wisdom behind it, it is among the most profound of yoga poses. Poses are not about performance; they are about experience. In this pose, one's hands are clasped, closing the circuitry of the heart energy. Also, one's two legs become like a single grounding rod, connecting with the earth. The upright plane between heaven and earth is divine. This is why humans among all creation have been gifted with upright posture. The more upright a creature is, the more aware it is. The most upright creature, humans, possess the potential of the greatest awareness—divine awareness. This divine plane, between heaven and earth, is occupied only by humans, upright cobras, and trees. It is the plane of kuṇḍalinī rising, of spiritual ascension, of touching the sky while rooted on earth.

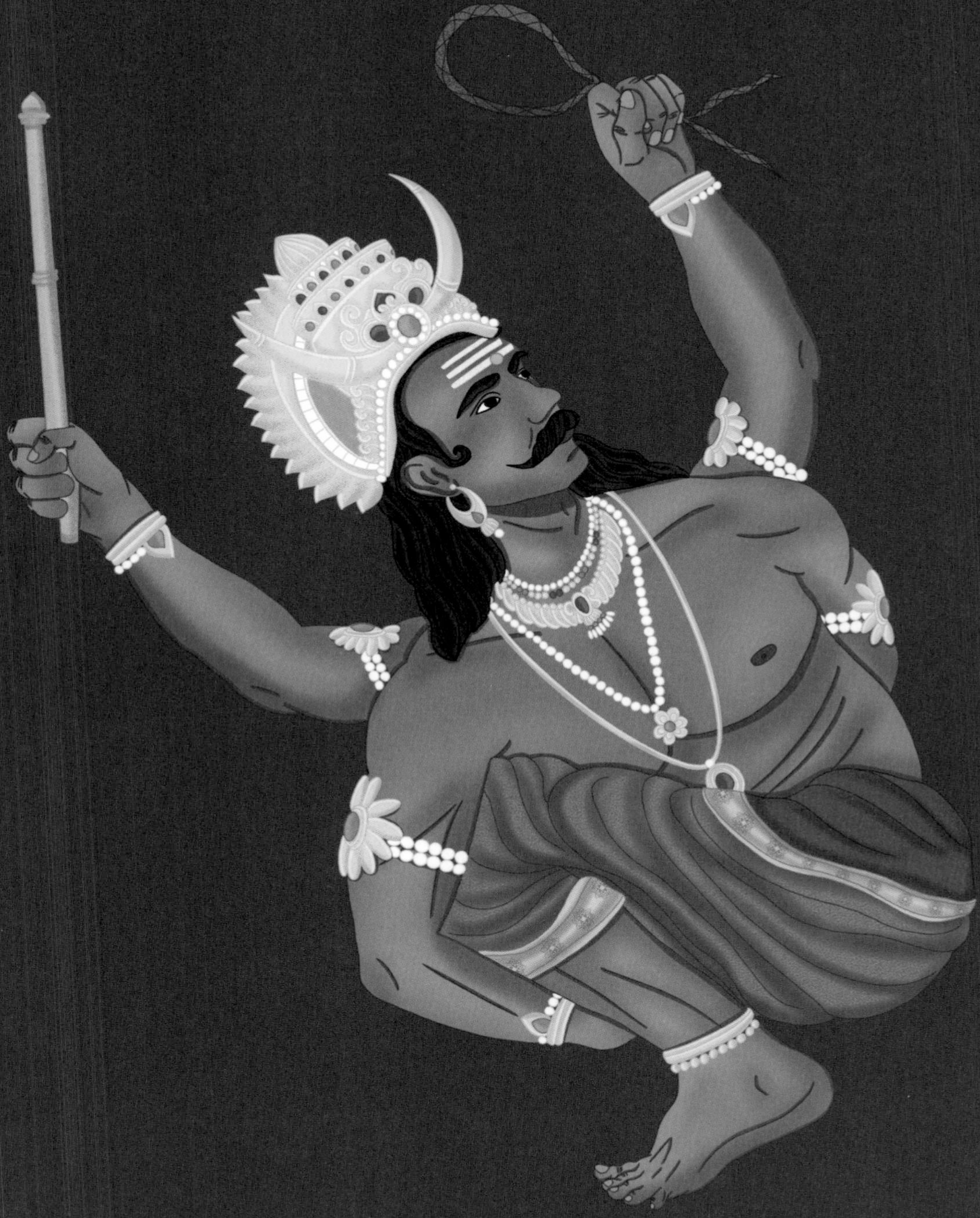

NOOSE POSE
PĀŚĀSANA

MĀRKAṆḌEYA'S MEDITATION

THEMES
Twisting
Agency
Surrender

ONCE THERE WAS A COUPLE WHO WERE CHILDLESS. In hopes of gaining a child, they took to worshipping the great god Śiva. One might ask why they might worship the Destroyer in order to create life, unless one understands that creation and destruction occupy two sides of the same transformation coin. The destruction of one thing necessarily entails the creation of another. And so, who better than Śiva to destroy the misery of their childless existence?

Day after day, the couple chanted the sacred syllables of the great god Śiva (oṃ namaḥ śivāya) with great earnestness and devotion until, pleased by their offering, the lord appeared before them to grant their boon. But, as is so often the case when the gods grant boons, there was a twist.

"I can indeed bless you with a child, my devotees. For the power of the gods not only carries out destiny, but can trump destiny, since we reside beyond the play of karma in our supreme state. I see that you both have enough merit in your karmic fields to have a child eventually, in a future life, but I will reshuffle the karmic debt, and bring him to you sooner, in this life. The only thing is you don't have enough merit to have a long-lived, noble son. So, I can bring you an ignoble dullard who will live 100 years, or a bright, pious, virtuous child who will live to only 16."

After a bit of deliberation, the couple agreed that they would much rather have a noble son for 16 years. And so, by Śiva's grace, the karmic deck was shuffled and a pious son was born to the couple. His name was Mārkaṇḍeya. Mārkaṇḍeya was prodigious in his intellectual and spiritual attainment, indeed the pride and joy of his family. He was already a full-blown sage by the time he turned 12. But as Mārkaṇḍeya's sixteenth birthday approached, he noticed that his parents rarely smiled, and teared up often. He suspected that they openly wept when he wasn't present. So, he confronted them about their grief. Then, breaking down, they let him in on the circumstances of his birth, confessing that they didn't anticipate how painful it would be to lose him so soon. Sage Mārkaṇḍeya responded:

"Mother, Father, weep not! Death is certain for all creatures, and you've made the right decision. An ounce of wisdom is worth a thousand years of ignorant toil. I shall take leave of you and go off to the forest to worship the great Śiva for the rest of my days. After all, I am grateful to him for summoning me to Earth in this life, that I may be raised by such loving parents."

Mārkaṇḍeya worshipped Śiva day and night. He crafted a Śiva Lingam, which he consecrated, establishing the energy of Śiva therein. He performed sacred rites to then holy Lingam, offering water, milk, honey, flowers, and flame, and chanted Śiva's sacred syllables all the while. As his hour of death drew near, Lord Yama appeared with his noose, to issue Mārkaṇḍeya's karma and usher him out of this life. Mārkaṇḍeya clasped the Lingam close to his heart, earnestly praying to Lord Śiva. Yama's noosed ended up encircling both Mārkaṇḍeya and the Lingam. Lord Śiva instantly appeared, declaring to Yama:

"Remove your noose from my Lingam, Lord Yama, for I am beyond the sway of time, and cannot possibly be trapped by karma."

Yama removed it instantly, realizing his unwitting insult. Yama muttered, "Forgive me, Lord. I merely meant to execute my duty to usher Mārkaṇḍeya out to this world as the sun is about to set on his 16th year."

Śiva beamed at Mārkaṇḍeya and replied to Yama: "The great sage was tested by my prophecy, and he has proven his worth. He shall attain immortal life, and remain 16 years old henceforth. The power of Śiva certainly trumps the power of death." With that, Yama bowed before the glorious Śiva and took leave of them both. Mārkaṇḍeya went on to illuminate the lost souls of the earth, forever young, and blessed by the power of Śiva.

The noose is the weapon of choice of for Yama, the god of death. It is his means of catching souls and taking them to the afterlife when their time on Earth is up. This is not a whimsical process. The grim reaper only arrives at the appointed hour, decided by the principle of karma. This is far too subtle and complex to be thought of merely in terms of simple fate. For, in light of the principle of karma, as you sow, so shall you reap. So, one's apparent destiny is the present result of one's previous free actions. One's span of life is delivered by destiny, but programmed by one's own actions. The grim reaper arrives at the appointed hour so that, for better or worse, you may reap what you have sown. Yama is a personification of this principle, and his weapon, the noose, represents the power of death as an instrument in one's own karmic ripening.

Karma is a profound and pervasive principle. It is the metaphysical corollary to Newton's third law of physics: for every action, there is an equal and opposite reaction. It is the principle that ensures we all receive our just deserts. But unlike actions in the material realm of physics, karma ripens in the spiritual realm of metaphysics which undergirds the mundane world we experience. When an apple is dropped, it falls immediately and predictably. But this is not the way of karmic apples, so to speak. When an act is undertaken, the opportune moment for its ripening may not arise for many years, or many lifetimes after. One may be now paying off a debt to someone in one's life that was incurred 10 lifetimes before. Similarly, one may have excellent luck in an area of life due to merit accumulated in a previous life. "Karma" refers not only to the metaphysical principle, but also the original act performed, and its result. The results of karma we experience as the power of destiny; our original actions we experience as free will. The noose represents the power of destiny to lock us into the fate we earned through our previous karmas. Yet grace can descend to alter one's karma.

Configured to emulate the knot and the function of the noose, this pose requires a great deal of rotation, as if one is rung out by the knots of karma. Surrender to the power of karma as destiny and embrace the power of dharma as free will. And summon grace to make the impossible, possible.

THUNDERBOLT POSE

VAJRĀSANA

WIELDING THE SECRET FIRE

THEMES
Concentration
Poise
Inner Power

THE PANTHEON OF VEDIC GODS is ruled by Indra, the thunderbolt-wielding king of heaven. Indra is preoccupied with power, and necessarily so, because his throne is much sought after, and needs to be defended at every turn. Beyond his personal desires, he has a divine duty to uphold. The gods of heaven need his leadership and protection, as do the rhythms of nature. He is the deity responsible for rain, storms, and thunder. Without him, the balance of weather on Earth would falter and nothing would grow.

Once, long ago, the great serpentine demon, Vṛtra, usurped the throne of Indra. At that time, chaos reigned in heaven as on earth. The gods were bereft of power, and the earth bereft of water. Vṛtra hoarded the heavenly waters, coveting them for himself and his kinsmen, not caring about the fate of the world. The earth grew dry and plant life withered. The animals were parched, and humans debilitated by drought. As much as it pained his pride, Indra knew he could not defeat this demon alone, so he ventured to the abode of Brahmā the Creator himself, for guidance on how to save creation.

"Hail Lord Brahmā!" began Indra upon entering. "You must assist us, Grandfather! My throne has been usurped by the serpent demon, Vṛtra, and he is keeping all the celestial

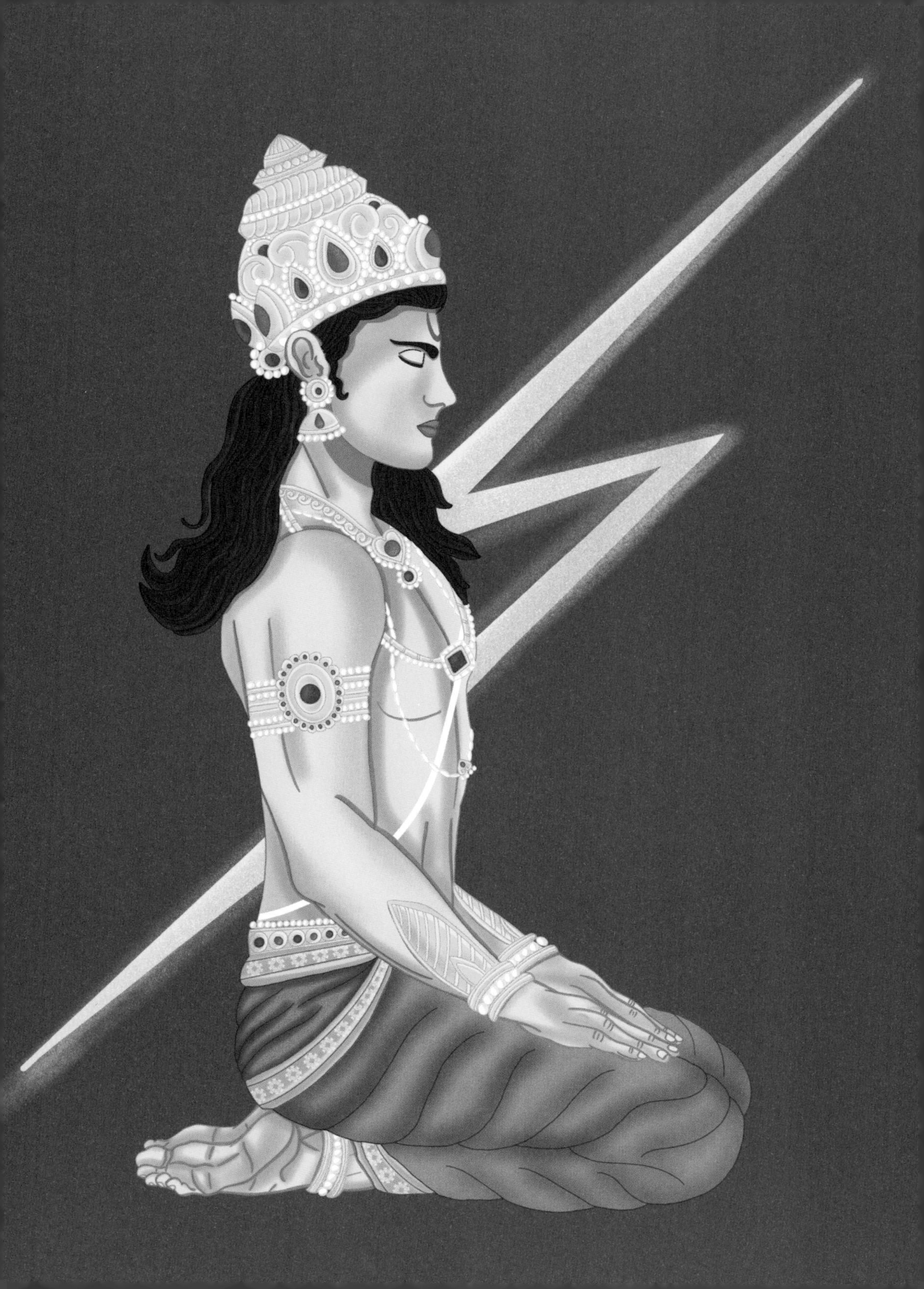

waters for himself! The gods are disenfranchised, and life on the earth is about to die out! Please tell me what weapons to wield against this formidable foe. He must be stopped!"

Lord Brahmā, stirred from his meditation, responded, "Indra, King of Gods, none of your weapons will work on this foe."

"How can you be so sure, Lord Brahmā?" asked Indra, dismayed.

"Because after Vṛtra performed a long penance, I granted him a boon. Like all demons, he sought immortality, and like always, I refused. So, he asked for the boon that no known weapon could kill him—a boon which I had no choice but to grant."

"All is lost!" cried Indra, devastated. "Thanks to your boon, he is invulnerable, Lord!"

"No creature in creation is completely invulnerable, King Indra. Everything that is born must die, for such is the way of things. You'll just need the right weapon to destroy him, and destroy him you shall."

"Right weapon?" Indra asked, confused. "Did you not say that you had blessed him such that no weapons could kill him?"

"Be calm, Indra, and hear my words. He was blessed such that no *existing* weapons could kill him. He's invulnerable to arrows, axes, maces, swords, and so on. So, all you must do is create a *new* weapon suited to the task!"

Indra's eyes seemed to open a little wider as the great Creator's plan began to dawn on him. "What kind of weapon must I make then? Surely he'd be invincible in the face of any blade I could forge."

"That is exactly why you will not be forging a blade," said Brahmā reassuringly. "Descend to Earth, to the Himālayan peaks. Find the great sage Dadhīchi who has garnered great power through many eons of yogic meditation. He will know what to do next."

Confused but intrigued, Indra did as he was told, and approached the abode of the great sage Dadhīchi. So abundant was his divine power that the very air around him seemed to hum with electric energy. Indra cautiously approached, trying to think of how exactly to politely interrupt the sage's profound penance.

But before he could, Dadhīci emerged from meditation and welcomed Indra with these words:

"Greetings King of Heaven. I know why you are here, and what must be done. I have accrued immense power through the raising of kuṇḍalinī in my subtle spine. This is the secret fire of creation that propels all things. This is the grace of the Holy Mother, the might of all creation. My time on Earth is done and now I know the purpose of the power which courses through my veins and pervades my very cells. I am to leave this world, leaving behind my energized body. From the bones of my spine, where the power is most concentrated, you will craft a weapon, the Vajra Thunderbolt, powered by the secret fire. No weapons made of material creation can compare to the divine power of kuṇḍalinī. Wield it well and accomplish your aim, King of Heaven."

Astounded and humbled, Indra bowed before the illustrious sage as he quit his body. He then took his energized remains to the divine craftsman Viśvakarman and asked him to forge the Vajra Thunderbolt, imbued with divine power by virtue of Dadhīci's penance. Thunder rolled and lightning cracked through the heavens as the great weapon was forged. The gods were in awe as their protector was granted this divine gift. The heavens and earth shook as Indra wielded the Vajra for the first time, and slew his enemy Vṛtra on the mountainside. The celestial waters were released and the Earth was hydrated again. The clouds of portent parted as the sun shone brightly to seal the triumph of Indra and the gods.

When sitting in thunderbolt pose, focus your attention on the body, and in particular, on your spine. Feel energy flow through you and understand that power divine prevails over all. Take inspiration from Dadhīci's dedicated penance, and allow the experience of this pose to afford an accumulation of divine energy in your own body. You wield your own Vajra in action, thoughts, and deeds. When your energy is raised, your very words hold power, and you will be able to accomplish your aims with relaxed poise and flowing grace.

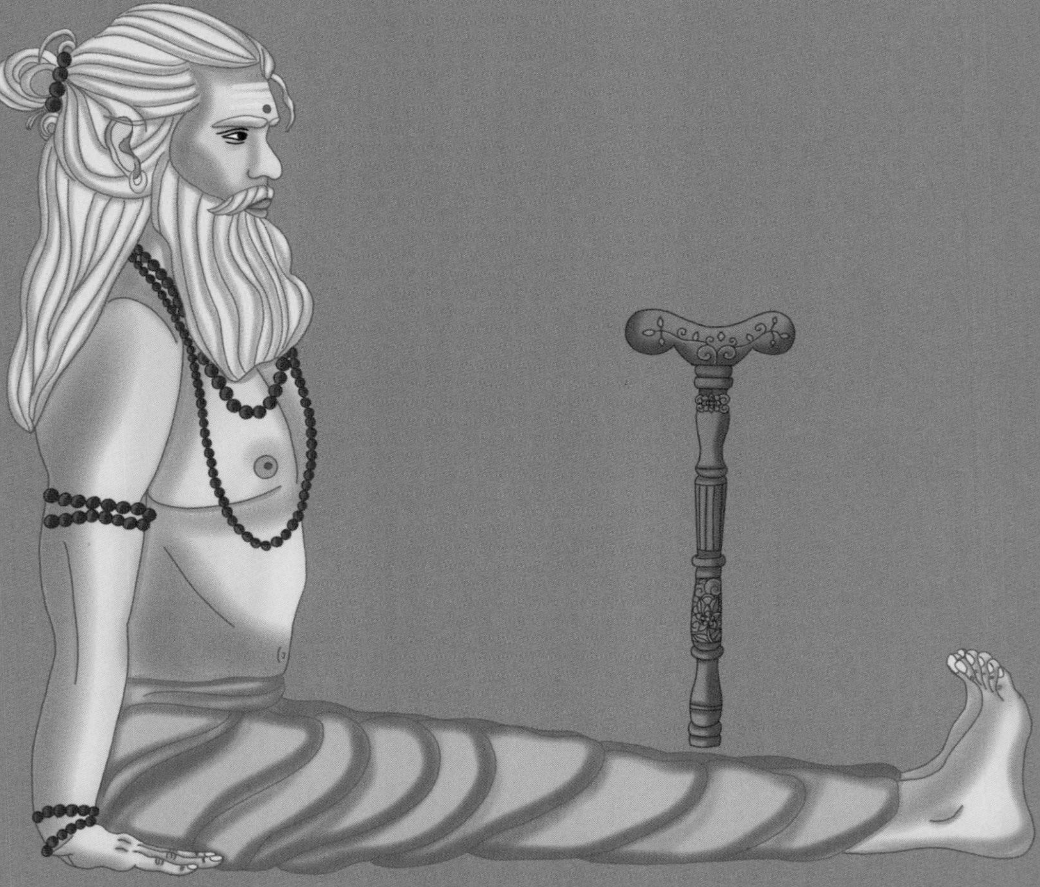

YOGIC STAFF POSE
YOGA-DAṆḌĀSANA

THE YOGĪ'S STAFF

THEMES
Strength
Straightening
Presence

ONCE, WHEN THE MIGHTY KING VIŚVĀMITRA was hunting in the forest, he came across the hermitage of the great sage Vasiṣṭha. The sage offered the king and his large entourage his hospitality. Viśvāmitra accepted, not expecting much from so humble a sage of modest accommodations. To his utter amazement, Vasiṣṭha served him and his entire retinue a sumptuous feast rivaling anything that could be served by even the palace kitchens with their full brigade of chefs. After all were sated, the king couldn't help but ask him how he had been able to produce such a feast. Vasiṣṭha informed him that it was quite simple, really. He was in possession of the great Cow of Plenty, Śabalā, who had emerged from the cosmic ocean, churned by the demons and gods when they were in search of the Elixir of Immortality. The cow was tended to by Vasiṣṭha, fed by his sacred rituals, and, in return, she provided for his needs. Though his needs were typically modest, this time he had needed a feast fit for a king, and she had happily obliged.

Enticed by the power he would wield were he to possess the Cow of Plenty, Viśvāmitra demanded that Vasiṣṭha hand her over immediately. Deferring to the authority of the king, sage Vasiṣṭha went out to fetch Śabalā, explaining the situation to her. "What can I do?" lamented Vasiṣṭha, "He is a great emperor, and I a lowly forest hermit. He has the power here, so I must part with you, my dear Śabalā." Śabalā's ears perked up, her tail twitched, and there was an indignant scowl upon her lips as she replied to Vasiṣṭha thus:

"Great sage! Know you not the power you possess? Yours is the power of the gods! It is by your divine power that I am nourished here, lest I perish. The king has only false power, an outer show, born of stealing the power of others! Own your power, Lord Sage! Give the command and I will destroy the pride of this wicked so-called king!"

Uplifted by Śabalā's invigorating counsel, Vasiṣṭha did just that, and Śabalā defeated Viśvāmitra and his army. Humiliated, but intent on possessing the Cow of Plenty, Viśmāmitra returned with an army of 10,000 men, complete with horses, chariots, elephants, and weapons of all kind. He was determined to storm Vasiṣṭha's ashram and steal the cosmic cow for himself. Sensing the army's approach, the sage went back to rouse Śabalā into action. He updated her on the colossal forces headed their way and urged her to be prepared to defend the ashram again.

The cow calmy replied, "Lord Sage, I will do no such thing."

Vasiṣṭha began panicking. "What do you mean, dear Śabalā, is all now lost? Will we not be able to defend against this rogue king and his army?"

Śabalā replied, "Of course we will, great sage, but by your own hand. Have you not been listening? You possess divine power within you, which comes from the gods. Spiritual power is far greater than martial power. Does kuṇḍalinī energy not course through your subtle spine? You don't need to develop a backbone; you already have one—a divine one at that! So, straighten yourself up and go defend your ashram!"

Energized by the words of the cow, and filled with righteous wrath, Vasiṣṭha went out to meet the oncoming army at the gate of his ashram. He had nothing more than his yogic staff with him, but he stood tall and faced King Viśvāmitra as he arrived at the head of his army.

Viśvāmitra began, "Feeble sage! You think your little cow can withstand the strength of 10,000 men? Before the day is out, I will have her squealing like a pig in meek surrender. Then she will see that her rightful place is by the side of a powerful king like myself."

"I do not need my dear Śabalā's help. It is by my divine power that she is nourished, and it shall be by that very power that you and this great army are defeated."

The king laughed in Vasiṣṭha's face, disbelieving that the sage could accomplish any such feat. But Vasiṣṭha simply raised his yogic staff to the heavens, and the lightning of the gods descended into it.

He centered himself and summoned all of the inner strength he could muster to wield the power of the gods. When he was ready, with a single flick of his yogic staff, waves of energy issued forth. Viśvāmitra's forces were all stunned, and fell to the ground. The horses and elephants bolted, maddened by the might of Vasiṣṭha's power. He then turned his staff to the flabbergasted Viśvāmitra and flicked it again. A bolt of energy knocked the king off his horse and brought him to his knees.

Vasiṣṭha went over to Viśvāmitra. Standing over him, he uttered these unforgettable words: "The duty of secular power is to protect spiritual power, whereby kingship is consecrated. When kings fail to do so, the gods themselves intervene. The power of a king is brittle, born of armies, pomp, and circumstance. But the divine power of the sage is eternal and far outlives the petty rise and fall of kings." Viśvāmitra relented and retreated once and for all. Understanding the true nature of divine power, he renounced his throne and retired to the forest to take up penance to Lord Śiva in the hopes of becoming a sage himself.

As you do this pose, straighten your spine, and sit erect. Feel the energy flowing through you. The upright plane is no mundane thing. Among all of the creatures upon the earth, only the human can inhabit it. It is a line of energy that connects the heavens and the earth. To cultivate this divine power, one needs guidance, discipline, and perseverance. The staff can represent the royal scepter, or a rod of discipline. But for the yogī, it represents the strength that is within the core of us all, and is just like that which was wielded by Vasiṣṭha through his yogī's staff.

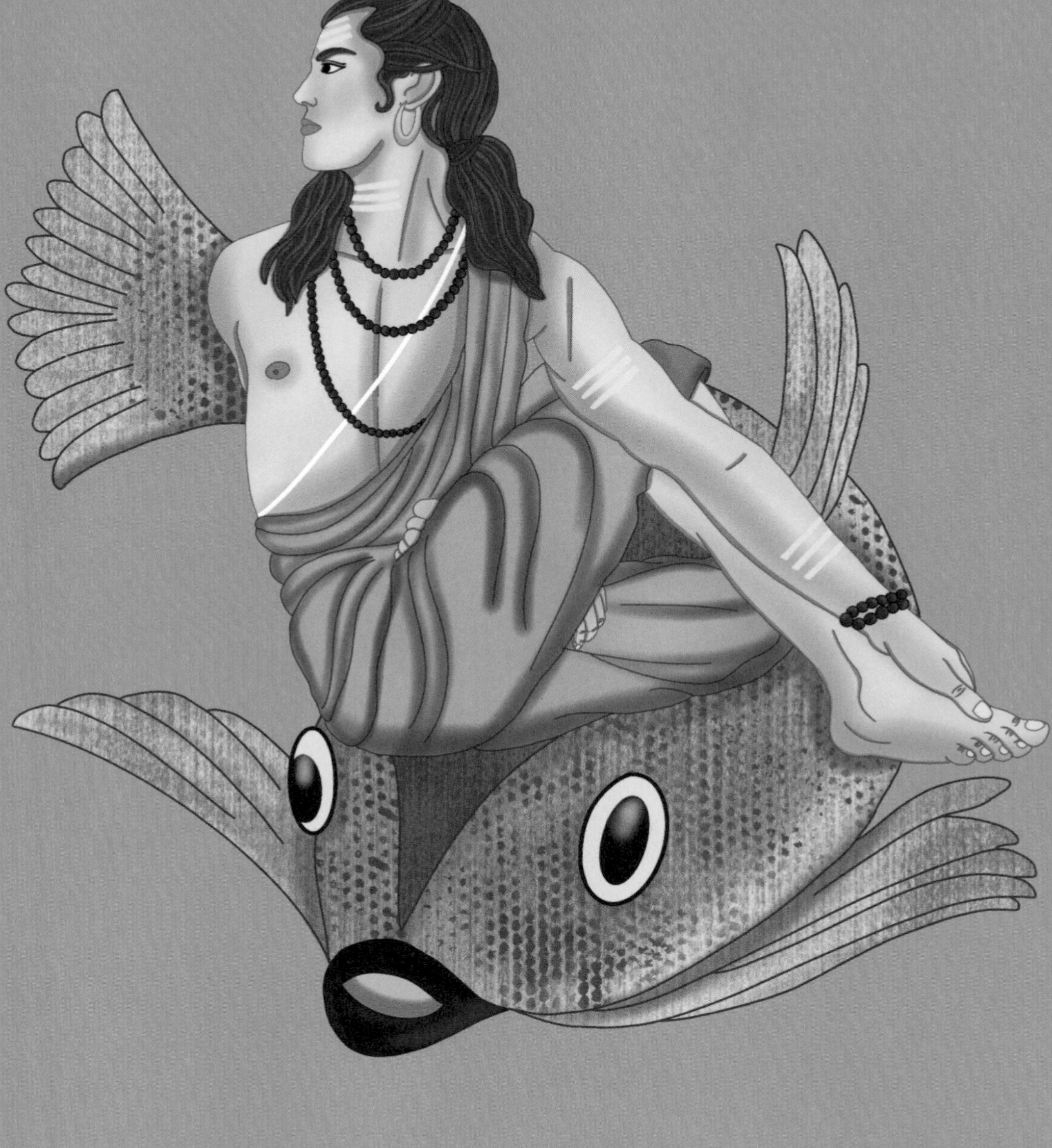

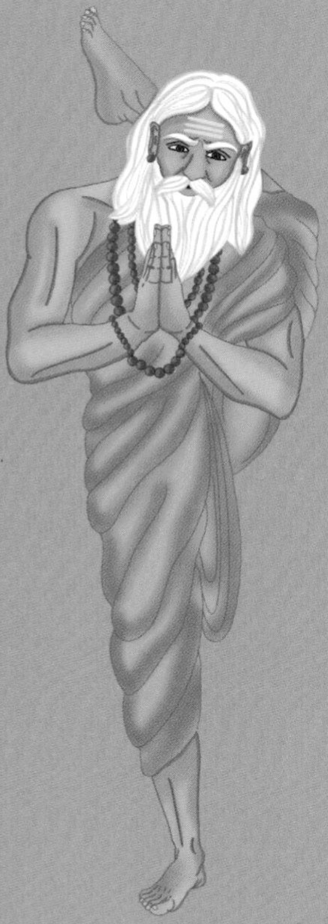

CHAPTER 5

The Wisdom of the Sages

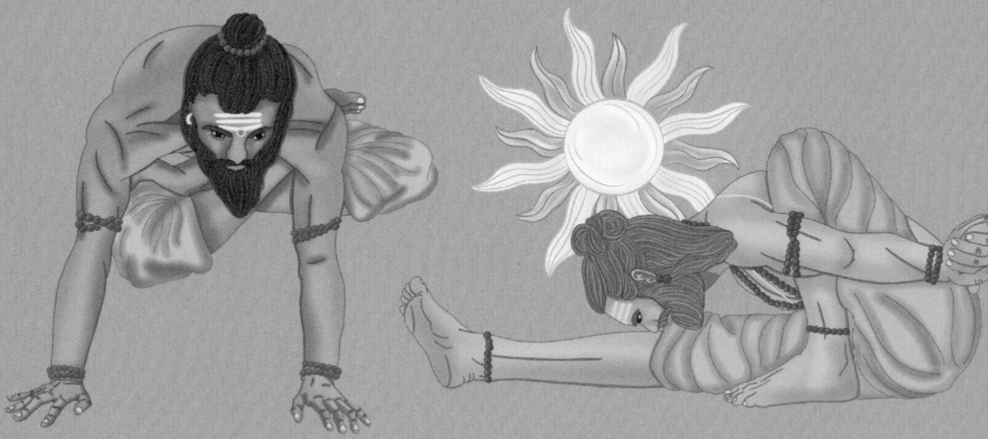

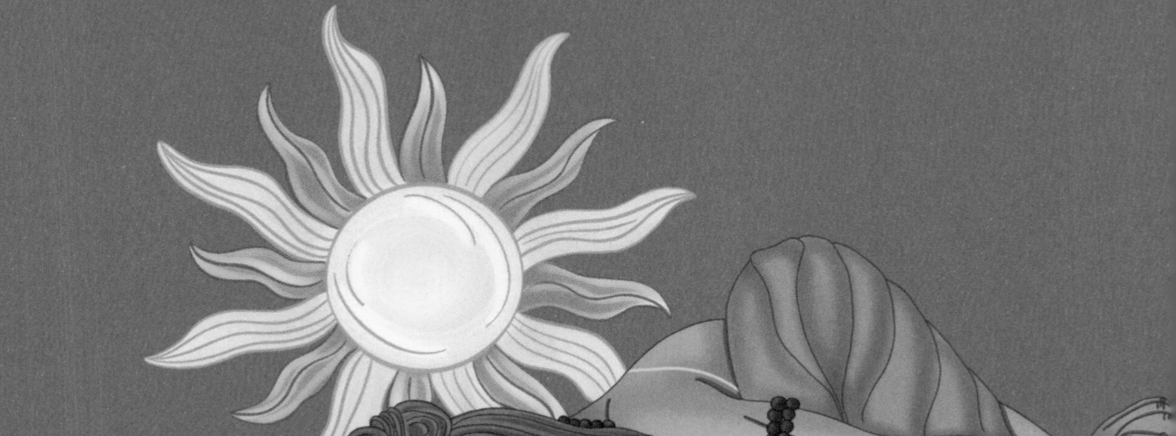

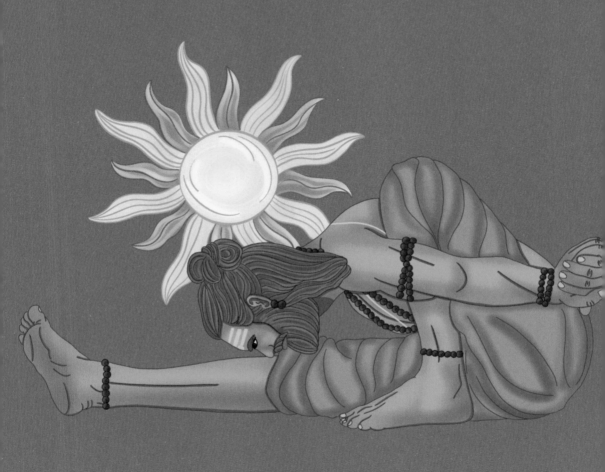

SAGE MARĪCI POSE

MARĪCYĀSANA

THE LEGACY OF LIGHT

THEMES
Lengthening
Stretching
Reverence

In the void, between creations, with nothing left over from the previous age, and nothing of the new one yet created, Viṣṇu the Preserver had nothing left to preserve. And so, he floated upon the oceanic abyss of pure potential, slumbering on his serpent couch. All had been returned back to this primordial state by Śiva's dance of transcendental bliss at the end of the previous age. All had been destroyed—dissolved back into this infinite ocean of pure potential. As Viṣṇu slumbered upon his serpent coach, Brahmā was again born from the lotus emanating from Viṣṇu's navel as he had been countless times before, and will be again in countless creations to come. For, existence is without beginning and without end, beyond limits imposed by reason, time, and space. These cycles of creation are not countless because we lack the ability to count them, but because they transcend the realm of counting itself. The concepts of measurement and quantification are simply irrelevant. The great galactic oceanic abyss is both the end of creation, and its beginning. It exists in infinity, beyond causation.

The newly born Brahmā gazed out upon the celestial abyss about him. He took an eternal moment to experience this time before time, to occupy this space beyond space, and mused to himself that the abyss before him was as utterly empty as any mind could imagine. And yet, when he considered its potential, the fullness of the abyss could not be doubted either! Lord Brahmā let out a deep and thunderous "oṃ", which rippled across the cosmic oceans, bringing into being the waves of time and space themselves. He went to work, orchestrating the symphony of sights and sounds that made up existence. He birthed the galaxies, stars, planets, and all that comprise the cosmos. He birthed too the physical and metaphysical principles by which the cosmos was bound, from gravity to the law of karma. Having completed his cosmic work, the Creator surveyed the cosmos and was pleased at what he saw. But now that the one had become many, separation and loneliness, too, crept into the consciousness of the Creator. So, as his final formal, act of creation, Brahmā brought forth seven beings, blessed sons, great sages all, born from his divine mind. Gifted with refined consciousness, Brahmā's sons became the Seven Seers of ancient India, versed in divine knowledge. Brahmā surveyed his work, looked upon his sons, and, satisfied, retired to his cosmic meditation.

Among Brahma's great and sagacious sons was the incandescent Marīci, whose name means "ray of light." His role in the universe was to dispel darkness on all planes by establishing a lineage that would enliven and illuminate the cosmos. This was Marīci's dharma. Through his illustrious lineage, Marīci would pass the light he received from Brahmā on to the world. Marīci had a great son named Kaśyapa, father of many classes of beings, including even Indra and the pantheon of the gods of heaven, and all their demon counterparts. All the subsequent warring between the children of Kaśyapa is nothing more than the play of dark and light, ultimately engineered to bring about the recognition and fostering of the light upon that particular plane of existence.

Kaśyapa was also the father of Sūrya, the sun itself. The celestial orb of the sun brings warmth and light to the world and is the giver of life on this planet. The sun is worshipped by millions, not only as the giver of life, but as emblematic of inner light—the light of consciousness that Sūrya inherited from his grandfather Marīci. Like his father Kaśyapa, the sun's tale, too, consists of the cosmic interplay between shadow and light.

Sūrya married the Goddess Saṃjñā, daughter of the great cosmic architect Tvāṭṛ—god of crafts and the divine artisan. Saṃjñā gave to Sūrya many important children, including Manu, the progenitor of all humankind of the present age, and Yama, God of Death. But over time, Sūrya's incandescence grew too much for Samjñā and she could not bear him. From her own shadow, she created a double of herself, named Chāyā. Sūrya was unaware of what had happened, and mistook Chāyā to be his wife, fathering another three children. Among them, another Manu, destined to be the progenitor of humanity in the next age; as well as Śani, the planet Saturn, and ruler of the principle of Karma. Eventually, Sūrya came to realise what had happened, and sought help from Saṃjñā's father Tvātṛ, who helped him to temper his great radiance, so that he and Saṃjñā could be reunited.

The legacy of the light of the illustrious Marīci, son of Brahmā, shines forth throughout creation, passed on to: his son Kaśyapa, father of beings, the demons, and gods; his grandson Sūrya, bringer of light; and Manu, progenitor of humankind. His was the spark of light from the Creator's consciousness which travelled through space and time to create the creatures of heaven and humanity itself.

In every case, it is the darkness, or the shadow, that affords the appreciation of the light, be it on the cosmic scale, or down here in the minutiae of our own experience. Sunlight, in isolation, without periods of darkness and shadow, would dry out the Earth, and render all the lands barren and burnt. Likewise, the conscious awareness of the mind that sunlight symbolizes cannot be switched on at all times.

This pose is quite profound. You are lengthening your spine, extending your being as you embody a ray of light. You are also strengthening and activating your core, your internal fire. And you are reverently bowing, grounding your energy with humility, as if you are a candle tipped over to kindle another, just like Marīci.

SAGE KAŚYAPA POSE
KAŚYAPĀSANA

KAŚYAPA, FATHER OF CREATURES

THEMES
Balance
Focus
Twist

Sage Kaśyapa was one of the Seven Sages of ancient India and a very important figure indeed. He had a very special role to play: he was the primary progenitor of various creatures. Upon wedding the 27 daughters of Dakṣa, Kaśyapa and his wives propagated many species. With his wife Vinatā, he fathered all avian creatures that take flight in the skies; foremost of these was the great Eagle Garuḍa. With his wife Kadrū, Kaśyapa fathered all of serpent kind, all that slithers upon the ground. Most famously, Kaśyapa is father to both the demons *and* the gods. He fathered the demons with his wife Diti (meaning division), and with his wife Aditi (meaning unification) he fathered the gods. Kaśyapa's innumerable progeny grace every crevice of creation with their colorful exploits. As vast as sage Kaśyapa's legacy is, his children were not exactly one happy family, in fact, their infighting is the stuff of many a great tale.

The most famous rivalry among them was between the demons and the gods. The demonic spawn of Kaśyapa and Diti were born first, and thus the elder. The gods, children of Kaśyapa and Aditi, though they were the younger, were able to trick them out of their share of the Elixir of Immortality. The gods used the demons to churn the cosmic ocean, but never delivered their share of the precious nectar, coveting it for themselves. By virtue of this ruse, the gods enjoy the

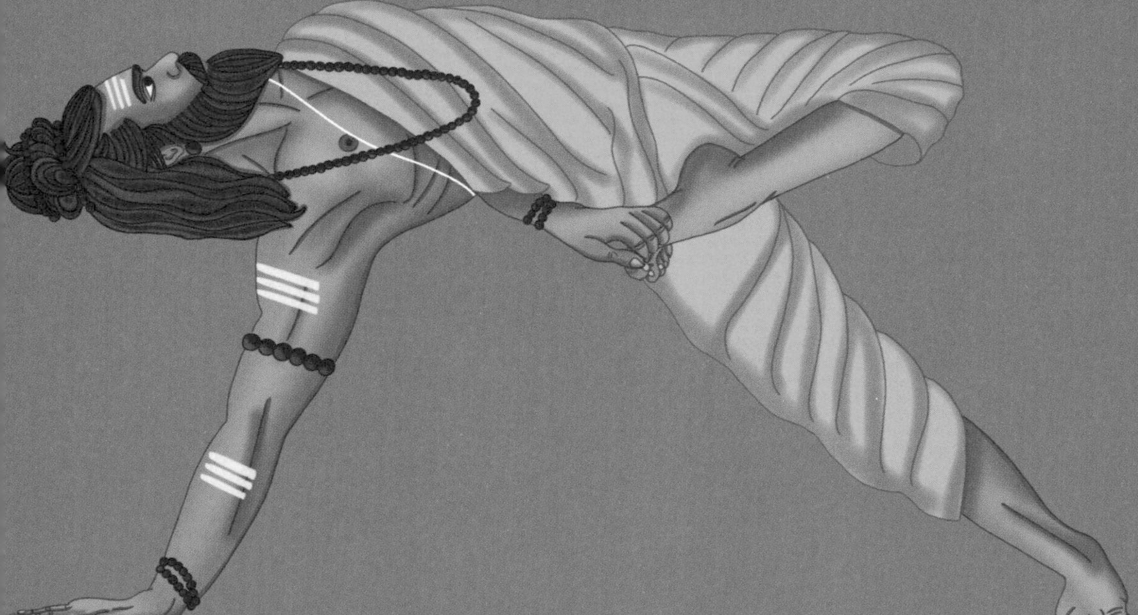

upper hand among all creatures fathered by Kaśyapa and his wives. What's a father to do in such a situation? Surely taking sides is not an option. So, Kaśyapa kept himself to himself, except on a few occasions where he couldn't help but be pulled this way or that by his children.

If the cosmic feud between the children of Diti and Aditi wasn't enough, a parallel feud raged on between his wives Vinatā, mother of birds, and Kadrū, mother of snakes. Despite the fact that these two classes of beings shared much in common, there was constant strife between them and they were always at odds. After all, birds eat snakes, and snakes eat the eggs of birds. Once, Kadrū went so far as to enslave her co-wife Vinatā through use of a clever bet. Garuḍa, the mighty eagle son of Vinatā decided to make a deal with the snakes:

"What it is it you serpents desire, in exchange for my mother's freedom?" he asked.

"We desire nothing from you, wretched bird! We have all we need, and besides, it gives our mother great pleasure to see yours enslaved. So, why should we seek to upset our own mother?"

"Surely you have your price, everyone does! Name it and it's yours!" heckled Garuḍa.

Upon reflection, the serpents thought up something they were certain Garuḍa could never procure: "The only thing that we would receive in exchange for your miserable mother's freedom would be the Elixir of Immortality! Fetch us the nectar and your mother shall be free!" hissed the snakes.

Garuḍa was astonished at their request, but quickly came to his senses, knowing they made it for the very purpose of dissuading him. A great being does not give up when they meet an obstacle. Rather than find an excuse to abandon their quest, they find a way to fullfill it. And the mighty eagle Garuḍa was cut from such a cloth. So, chest puffed out, spine straight, he defiantly chirped to the serpents assembled, "So be it! Your scheme will backfire, for I *will* procure the elixir for you, and my mother *will* be free, as sure as the sun rises in the East!"

Garuḍa went to visit his mother in captivity to seek her blessings, and her advice on how to proceed.

"My son," replied Vinatā, "what you seek to do is impossible. The elixir is most precious to the gods and they guard it well. But if anyone can make the impossible possible, you can. My instinct tells me that you should go and see your father, and seek his aid. Godspeed, my son!"

Garuḍa was wary of his mother's counsel. He knew that Kaśyapa never got involved in his children's feuds. After all, he was father to all of them! Nevertheless, Garuḍa flew to the peaks of the Himālayas, where his father was practicing austerities. Once there, he explained how Vinatā had been enslaved by Kadrū, mother of snakes. He also relayed news of the deal he had made with the snakes, and pleaded for Kaśyapa's help.

"What you seek is impossible, dear Garuḍa, my son. Moreover, I do not get involved in my children's unending squabbles. It would drive any father mad, even a sage like me, born of Brahmā himself!"

"Father, there is time for forbearance and time for action. Inaction in the face of dire need, too, is a decision you make, and with it comes consequences. Does the ill karma of a wife enslaved truly befit you, great father, Kaśyapa, son of Brahmā?"

Reflecting on Garuḍa's words, Kaśyapa knew them to be wise. He recognized that inaction in the face of oppression is itself an action that would yield karmic consequences just like any other. With that realization, he whispered the secret into Garuḍa's ear about the vulnerability of the gods, and the exact manner in which he would be able to wrest some ambrosia from them. No living mortal knows the secret Kaśyapa whispered to Garuḍa, lest they, too, use it to procure the elixir. To the astonishment of the serpents, Garuḍa was able to procure them some elixir and free the mother of birds, Vinatā, thereby. And Kaśyapa learned a very valuable lesson about inaction, responsibility, and the power of karma.

This posture requires great balance and focus. Also, it is one which pulls you in different directions, much as Kaśyapa is pulled by the creatures he spawns. Stay steadfast in your stance, but flexible as well. One part of you may well relish remaining in lotus and meditating undisturbed, but as yogī, you need to combine this with "taking a stand." As with this posture, you're called to find poise in life's trials and tribulations, navigating them with wisdom in action.

SAGE ṚCĪKA POSE

ṚCĪKĀSANA

THE INVERSION OF SAGE AND KING

THEMES:
Balance
Stability
Inversion

THE GREAT KING GĀDHĪ lived a pious life in the forest with his beautiful daughter Satyavatī. When Satyavatī came of age, the great sage Ṛcīka asked for her hand in marriage. Satyavatī was quite keen on marrying the exalted sage. Who wouldn't want so wise and noble a husband? King Gādhī consented to their union, on the condition that the sage prepared a potion so that his own wife could conceive a great warrior. "Certainly, noble king," replied Ṛcīka, "I can surely prepare such a divine concoction for your wife. I will also prepare one for your daughter, Satyavatī, whereby she will conceive, since I am committed to celibacy, as it is the path to divine truth." The king and his wife were delighted, as was Satyavatī. Their marriage was set.

One night soon after the wedding, the sage retired to his sacred space and prepared two bowls of porridge upon which he performed powerful rituals, reciting secret Sanskrit mantras over each bowl in turn. The next morning, he presented the delighted Satyavatī with the two bowls of porridge and explained which one was for her, and which for her mother. Satyavatī excitedly paid him heartfelt thanks, and skipped off to her mother so that they may partake in their divine porridge together. Satyavatī presented her mother with her porridge, and she too, was overjoyed. She was of an ancient royal house, and success and prestige were

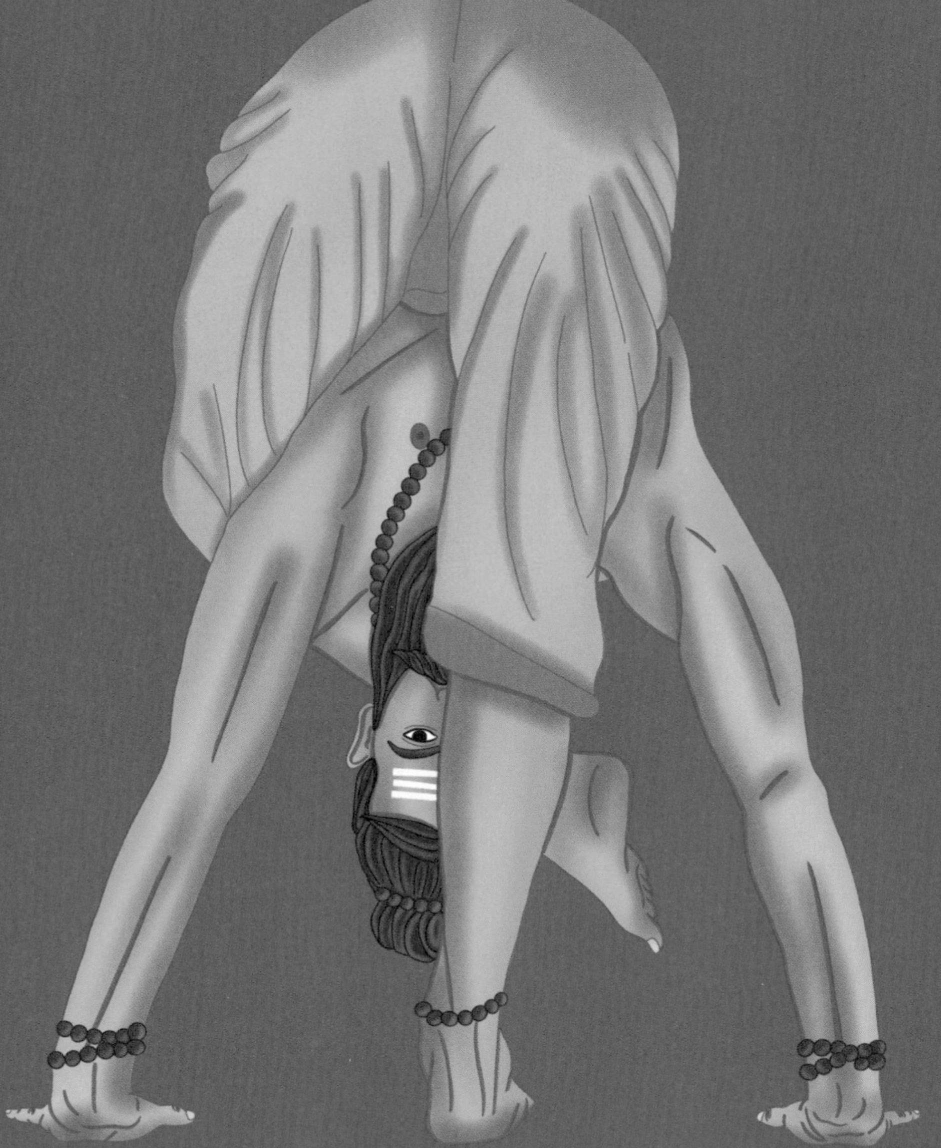

important to her. She wanted the best! Figuring that the sage would obviously save the best for his wife, and give the second best to his mother-in-law, she swapped the bowls of porridge while Satyavatī wasn't looking. After eating the divine porridge, Satyavatī returned to Ṛcīka, her face radiant with the child she now carried growing inside her. Upon entering their forest hut, she beamed her illustrious husband a radiant smile, evidencing her successful conception. Ṛcīka, delighted to see her, returned her smile. But a moment later he turned ashen, shocked as his advanced powers of perception afforded him some idea of what had happened.

"What is it, beloved?" asked Satyavatī, slightly alarmed. "Did the porridge not take? I definitely feel changed, and can sense a child growing within me."

"Yes, it definitely took, my dear Satyavatī, for you are radiant with child! But did you take the porridge I gave you, or did you consume the one I specified was for your mother?"

"These divine potions known to you sages are definitely beyond me, and I would never meddle with them. I gave my mother the one you specified was hers, and kept the one you specified was mine, my Lord. What is the issue?"

Ṛcīka took a moment to close his eyes and focus his inner sight. He then saw what had happened: his mother-in-law had switched the porridges! "My dear Satyavatī, thinking her concoction inferior to yours, your ambitious mother switched them, unbeknownst to you! I infused your mother's potion with the qualities of a warrior, as per your father's request. Hers was to have been a child befitting a great royal house. In your potion, I infused the qualities of a brahmin: compassion, gentleness, purity, truth. But now, your royal mother has conceived a Brahminic child, and you, my dear, have conceived a great warrior!"

"Dear Ṛcīka, best of sages, surely there is something you can do!" exclaimed Satyavatī, shocked."I would love nothing more than to bear you a brahminical son, befitting a sage as exalted as yourself! Could you perhaps defer the effects of the potions for a generation so that I could bear you a wise and sagacious son, and my mother birth a fierce warrior?"

Ṛcīka was able to grant Satyavatī's wish, and they brought forth another great sage, Jamadagni. Jamadagni's son, Paraśurāma, however, though born and raised a brahmin, became a powerful warrior indeed. Likewise, due to the porridge exchange, Satyavatī's royal mother gave birth to King Viśvāmitra, a fierce warrior who eventually abdicated his throne and undertook great penance so that Śiva would grant him the boon of being transformed into a contented sage. Paraśurāma and Viśvāmitra were inverse versions of each other: the former was born a brahmin, but adopted the ways of the warrior, while the second was born a warrior and king, yet adopted the ways of a sage.

This pose involves a deep inversion, much like the story. Yet, also like the story of Ṛcīka, you need to stay grounded with a single foot firmly planted on the ground. You also need to balance your weight between two hands, which represent the two types of power discussed in the story. The brahmin's power is concentrated in the great sages of ancient India. The warrior's power finds its apex in the king. These two manifestations of—one outer, physical, secular; the other inner, spiritual, sacred—need to be brought into balance. They complement each other. And so, the story of Ṛcīka is the story of the reversals of the power roles of sages and kings, one which required great grounding and balance to succeed.

SAGE VASIṢṬHA POSE

VASIṢṬHĀSANA

VASIṢṬHA, BEST OF SAGES

THEMES
Focus
Forbearance
Strength

Once, the mighty King Viśvāmitra was hunting in the woods, accompanied by a royal entourage of grand proportions, as befitting such a king.

While deep in the woods, they came across the quaint hermitage of a great sage named Vasiṣṭha. Vasiṣṭha was one of the original Seven Sages of ancient India, spawned by the Creator Brahmā himself. He was, in fact, the very greatest of sages, versed in Vedic learning as well as advanced spiritual attainment. He had perfected the virtues of humility, nonviolence, forgiveness, restraint, and compassion. Beyond being an ascetic adept, he was also the best of brahmins, a high priest, and well versed in social etiquette. He well understood the crucial interplay between brahmins—holders of spiritual knowledge—and kṣatriyas —warriors, administrators, rulers, and holders of social office. Embodying the ancient Sanskrit dictum that "the guest is God," Vasiṣṭha graciously greeted the mighty king, shining like the midday sun by the power of his ascetic practices. The humble sage offered to water and feed the ruler and his entire retinue. Viśvāmitra graciously accepted, not expecting too much given the sage's modest abode. It would be a feat to feed an entourage that size, even for the palace dining hall!

After taking a bit of time to make the necessary preparation, the brahmin sage invited the king and his royal

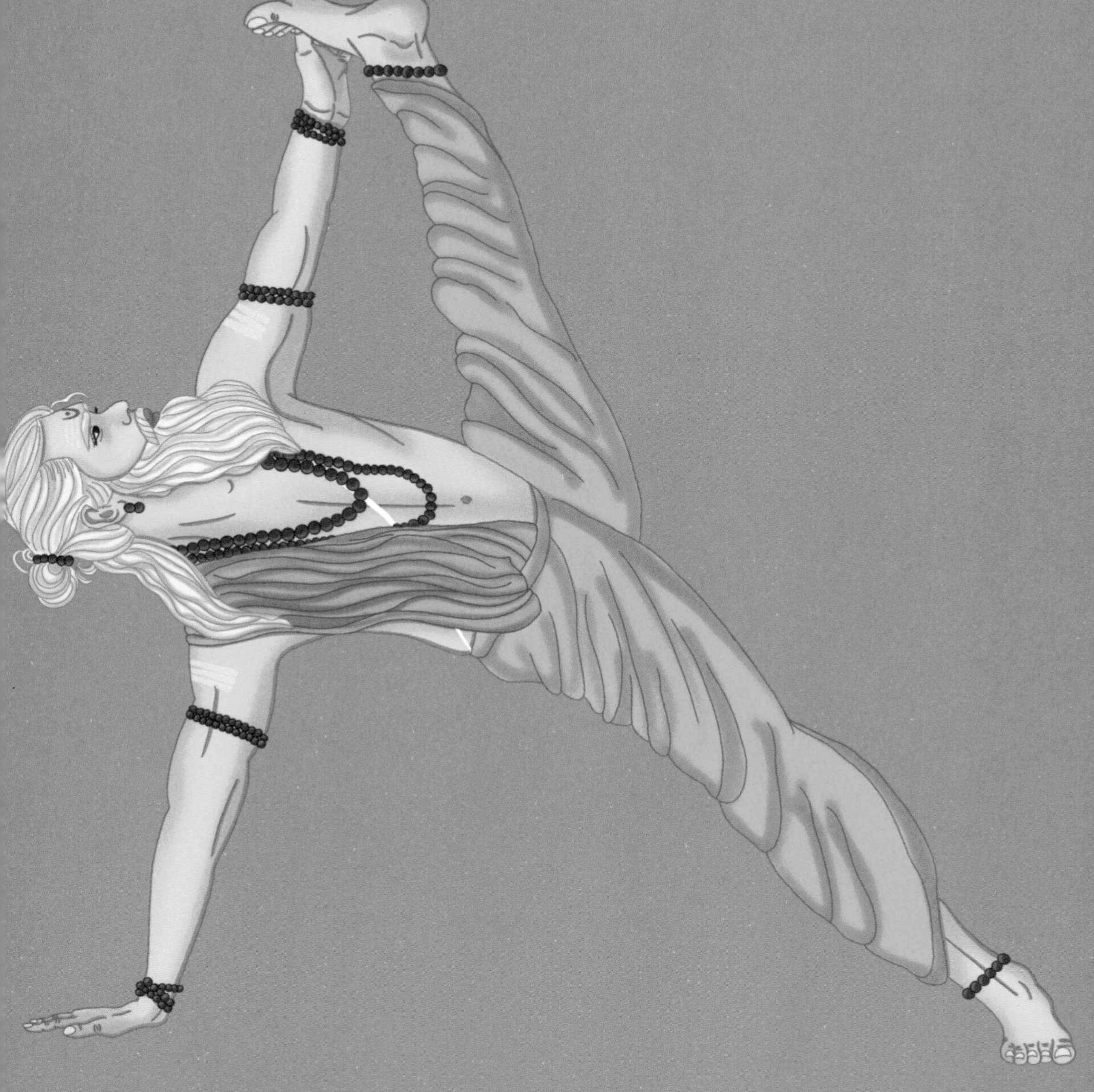

retinue into the hermitage. To the astonishment of all, the guests were greeted with an array of sumptuous food and drink of epic proportions. Mouthwatering dishes were served in lavish style, and all ate their fill. When they were finished, Viśvāmitra expressed his gratitude, to which Vasiṣṭha replied: "Mighty king, devouring food is akin to the sacred fire devouring sacrificial offerings. So, the sacrifice of hospitality is offered unto the internal fire of one's guests. So, I am delighted to hear you are so well sated! My sacrifice has been accepted."

The king's curiosity overcame him. "Surely a man of your spiritual stature lives modestly," he asked, "and yet it seems your hermitage is stocked with the finest of foods in lavish supply! How could this be?"

"Great king," responded the sage, "you are right that I live humbly in the material world. My riches are spiritual. But behind my hermitage dwells Śabalā, the great wish fullfilling cow, who provides for my needs in return for the spiritual practices I perform for her care."

The king had heard tell of the legend of Śabalā, the magical cow that had emerged from the cosmic ocean in ancient times, but he never imagined that he might stumble across such a creature within the bounds of his own kingdom! A powerful temptation arose in him, and his eyes glazed over as he fantasized about what he could do with such a possession. Visions of endless finery, weapons, riches, and treasures began to fill his mind, and he began to salivate. All gratitude and humility were forgotten, their place taken now by insatiable greed and pride.

"Why would so powerful a creature belong to so lowly a forest ascetic, brahmin?" he sneered. "Technically, I possess all that rests within my realm, so the cow is mine! I therefore command you to hand her over to me immediately!"

"Mighty king," pleaded the sage, "you misunderstand. The cow does not *belong* to me, or anyone for that matter! Like the sun, moon, and stars, she is free. She was merely placed in my care. It is my divine rituals that nourish her. She provides only for my needs in return. While my needs are generally modest, I needed a feast to offer the hospitality befitting you and your entourage, and so she provided one. She is not mine to give, nor can she thrive without the spiritual power generated by my rituals."

"You dare to refuse your king? You no doubt wish to keep her for yourself! I don't need your consent to take her, for you stand no chance against my powerful forces."

Despondent and dismayed, the sage went off to fetch Śabalā, hunched over with resignation. He explained the situation, concluding, "what can I do but comply? I am no match for the king and his army, who are now strong and well fed thanks to your grace."

"Brahmin sage, hear my counsel!" declared the cosmic cow. "The king possesses no true power, for his is merely bestowed by his army and his subjects. Political power is moored to this decaying outer world, but ours is the power of the gods. Divine power emerges from the eternal, the real, the true. The sage is far more powerful than the sovereign. Just wish it so, O mighty man, and I shall use this divine power to crush the pride of this wicked king."

Heeding the wisdom of Śabalā, the sage, with a twinkle in his eye, commanded the cow to slaughter the pride of the sovereign. The sage led the cow to the king, but the king could not budge her, and nor could any of his entourage. Viśvāmitra left the heritage, tail between his legs, his pride crushed.

According to Indian philosophy, all of creation consists of three modes: sattva *(goodness, lightness, clarity),* rajas *(passion, drive, energy) and* tamas *(heaviness, darkness, inertia). This applies to states of consciousness as well as inanimate things. Vāsiṣṭhāsana (side plank) is born of sattva, i.e., purity, lightness, goodness, clarity. Sage Vasiṣṭha predominantly operates within the mode of sattva. As such, this is the mode that this āsana cultivates. However, the story of Vasiṣṭha is the story of sattva with a twist of rajas. Vasiṣṭha is gracious and content, yet needs to adopt passion to defend his divinity, and that of Śabalā, the wish-fullfilling cow, from exploitation. This pose represents and enacts the balancing act of self-seeking spiritual consciousness in a mundane, self-serving world. It requires focus, forbearance, and inner strength.*

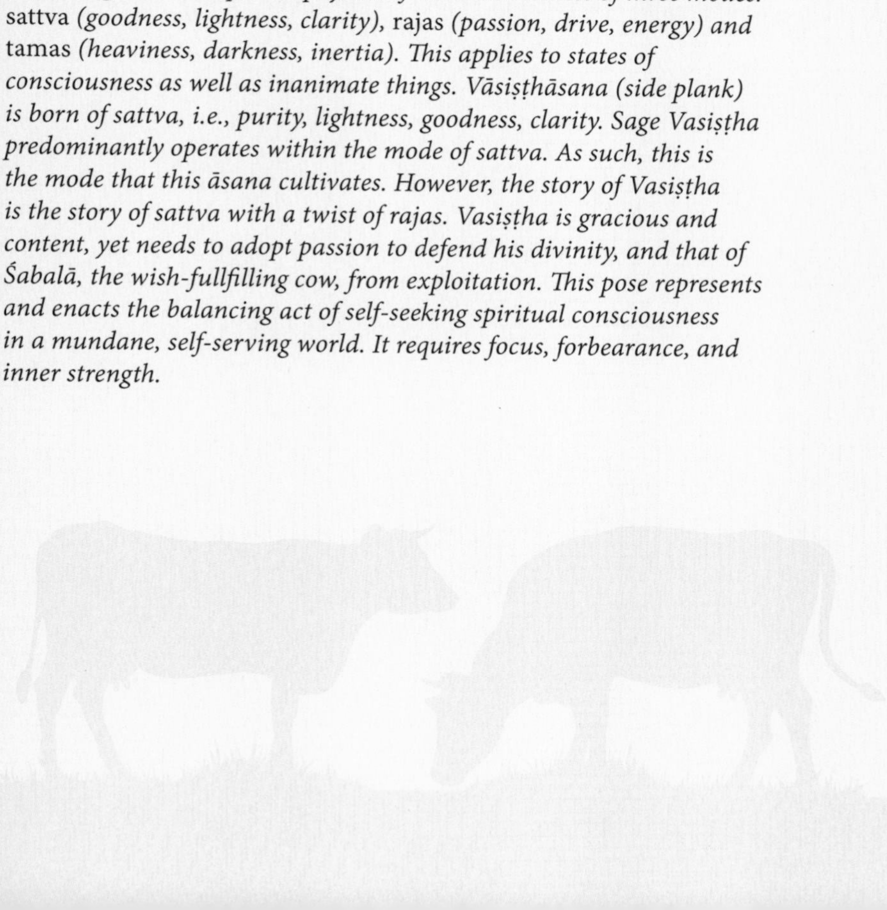

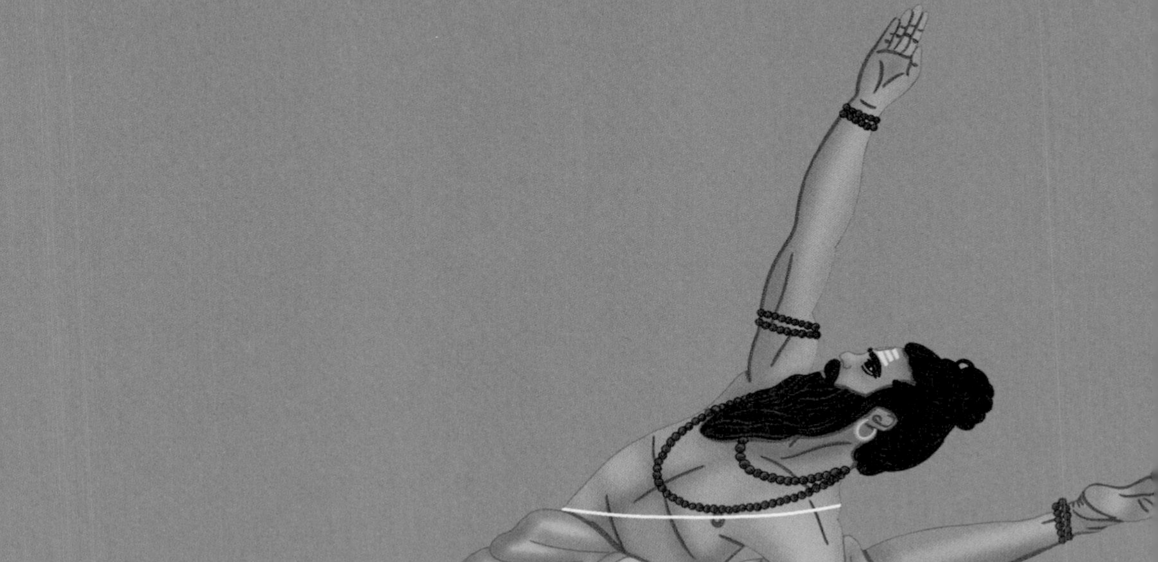

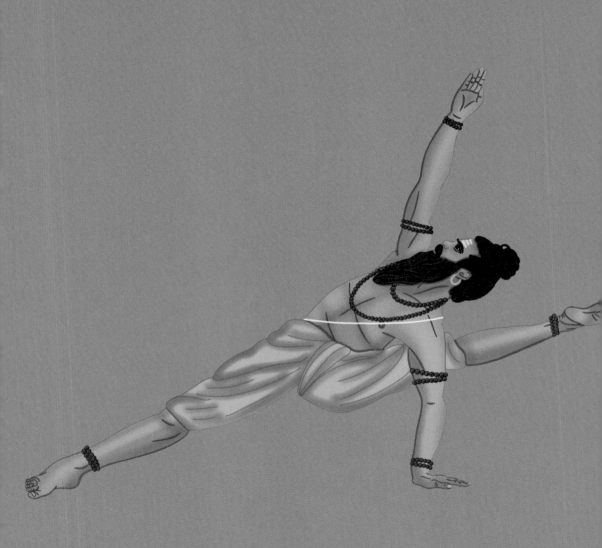

SAGE VIŚVĀMITRA POSE

VIŚVĀMITRĀSANA

VIŚVĀMITRA, THE ROYAL SAGE

THEMES
Focus
Determination
Discernment

ONCE, WHILE HUNTING IN THE FOREST, the mighty King Viśvāmitra and his grand entourage came across the hermitage of the great sage, Vasiṣṭha. The sage extended his gracious hospitality to the king and his royal retinue, miraculously producing a feast in the blinking of an eye. Once sated, the king couldn't help but ask just how the sage was able to accomplish this feat. Vasiṣṭha explained that behind his hermitage dwelt the divine wish fullfilling cow, Śabalā. Coveting the cow for himself, the king ordered the sage to fetch her. But once he did, the cow would not budge. Even the strength of the king's entire army was no match for this single celestial cow. So Viśvāmitra left the hermitage humiliated by sage Vasiṣṭha, having tried in vain to take Śabalā from him.

Determined to defeat the sage, Viśvāmitra left his heir in charge of the kingdom and retired to the forest to undertake penance to Lord Śiva. After worshipping the Lord of Yogīs with steadfast devotion for many years, Śiva appeared before the king and granted him a boon. "Great Śiva, you are the most powerful of all gods! Surely you know the ways of strength. As you no doubt perceived through your third eye, my forces were insufficient to contend with Vasiṣṭha's cow! So, great god, I wish for more forces. Increase my army a thousand-fold, and make my warriors indefatigable!"

Śiva, smiling mysteriously, granted his wish. "You shall attain the power you seek, King Viśvāmitra! Your forces will increase a thousand-fold, and be populated by men of unlimited stamina. So be it!" Then he vanished.

Delighted at having received his wish, Viśvāmitra, accompanied by his martial hordes, descended upon Vasiṣṭha's hermitage, intending to storm it and steal Śabalā away for himself. Standing confidently at the head of his formidable army, the puffed-up king commanded, "Come out and face me you cowardly sage! You are about to learn what power a king wields!"

The sage emerged, contented, shining like the midday sun, ablaze with the energy of his spiritual practices. He recalled how disempowered he felt when the king was last there, and how willing he was to give his power away to this tyrannical man. He recalled the wise counsel of his beloved cow, nourished by the divine power of his sacred rituals. The cow had counselled that while a king wields outer, social power, a sage wields divine, inner power. The king's power is born of time and circumstance, while the sage's power is imperishable. Knowing all this, the sage stood resolute and faced the king. Standing up straight with his staff at his side, the sage declared:

"Behold, I stand before you, ready to face you and your army. My fear has been dispelled by discernment. I see clearly now who is more powerful! Let us test the might of your army, shall we? There can be no comparison between mere martial might of an earthly king, and the colossal cosmic power of a brahmin sage. Behold as I smite you with the power of the gods!" With this, Vasiṣṭha raised his hermit's staff to the heavens and it was filled with the divine power, emitting bolts of lightning. Then he turned it upon the forces before him. By wielding the divine power, the sage annihilated the King's vast forces with a single stroke of his staff.

Viśvāmitra retreated, astonished, afraid, and utterly demoralized. Twice now, he had been brought to his knees by the sage. With a clouded mind, he turned, once again to penance. He sat in lotus posture, focused his mind on Śiva's divine form, and chanted his sacred syllables. He went without food and water, and focused only on the lord. His great penance lasted a thousand years. The Lord of Yogīs appeared then before him with a knowing smile, asking, "Since the forces with which I blessed you last were insufficient to combat the sage, then I suppose you now seek an even greater force with which to overcome him? Perhaps one thousand times again the size and strength?"

But this time the king had been humbled by his penance, so he bowed before the lord and said, "Great Śiva, Lord of Yogīs, I now know that weapons of this world are no match for yogic power. For might is material, divinity everlasting. The issue in my confrontation with the great sage Vasiṣṭha was not in the mere *quantity* of my forces, but in their *quality*. Through my centuries of meditations upon your divine form, I realize that your great power comes from within, not without. I no longer wish to conquer Vasiṣṭha, or anyone, for that matter! Instead, I wish to become a brahmin sage myself. I wish to know true power. Grant me the divine insight needed to purify my ego and learn life's mysteries. Grant me the power of the sage, Great Lord! For this, I sacrifice all of my earthly status and riches." Sensing Viśvāmitra's sincerity, Śiva granted this most precious of boons. For the first and last time in history, a king was transformed into a sage.

Vasiṣṭha and Viśvāmitra represent crucial aspects of the human experience. The great sage represents our capacity to learn, discern, and grow wise. He represents the inner life, and all of the wish fullfilling riches that such divine power alone can bring. The king represents our command of the outer life, our ability to rise through the ranks and wield social power. He is our drive to have, and to be, more than we are. The first impulse is born of sattva, and prioritizes the spiritual. The second is born of rajas, and prioritizes the social.

Both Vasiṣṭhāsana and Viśvāmitrāsana involve a balancing act. While the king still desires power, his desire has been sublimated to the realm of spiritual power. Rather than martial force, he is called to mystical forces. This pair of poses represents the interplay between two types of power: inner and outer, worldly and otherworldly, social and spiritual. Like Vasiṣṭhāsana, Viśvāmitrāsana entails balance and poise, but it also involves more external pressure. It activates the quality of rajas, that is, heat, ambition, passion, and drive.

Like Viśvāmitra, one needs to be firmly planted in one's standing. One needs to perform penance, twisting oneself not out of shape, but into another shape, all the while gazing upwards toward the heavens. The grace and poise attained by Viśvāmitra entail a great deal of effort and purification. This pose requires dynamism and dedication, combining standing, twisting, hip opening, and arm balance all in one. Viśvāmitra's story, along with his pose, reminds us that persistence, perseverance, dedication, and focus pay off to make the impossible, possible.

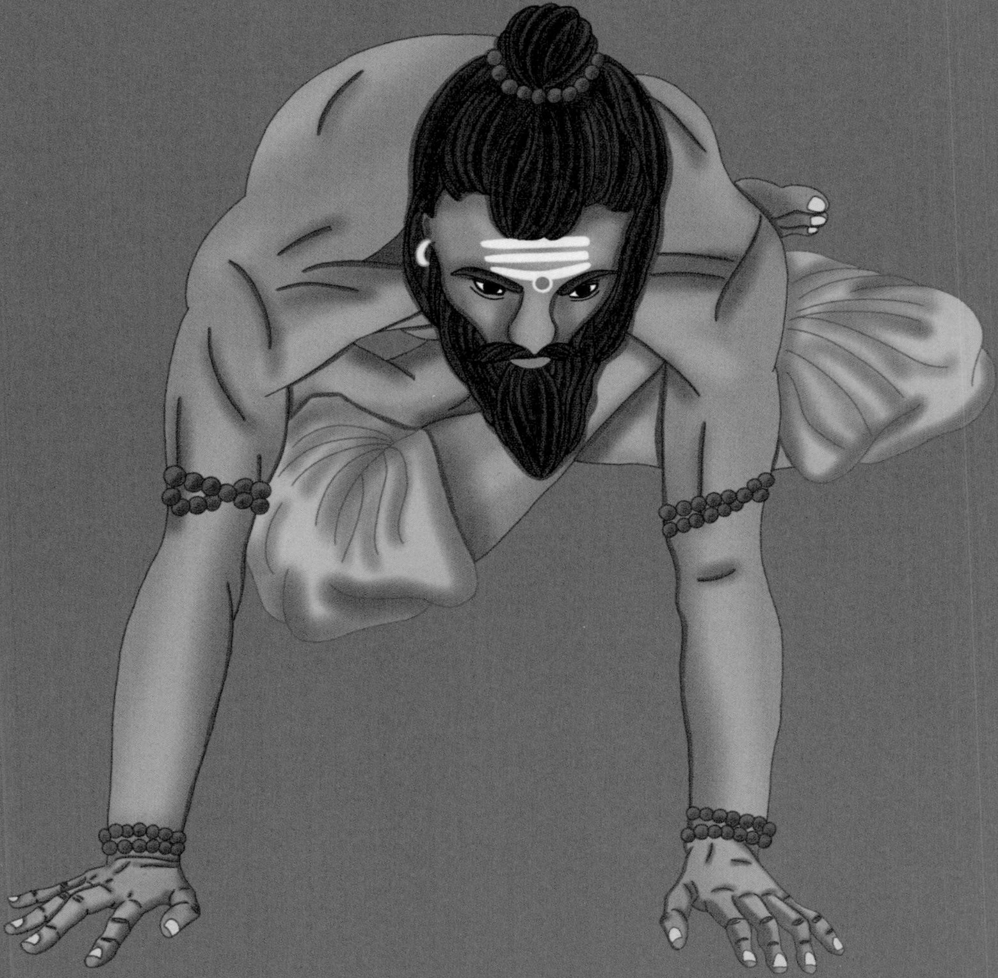

SAGE GĀLAVA POSE
GĀLAVĀSANA

WHITE HORSES WITH BLACK EARS

THEMES:
Commitment
Perseverance
Strength

There was once a devoted pupil of the great sage Viśvāmitra named Gālava. The day came when Gālava was set to graduate from his studies after years of training. It was customary at this time for students to offer a ritual fee of the teacher's choosing as a token of appreciation for their years of unrelenting tutelage and care. Upon being asked what ritual fee he desired, Viśvāmitra replied that he was content and needed nothing. But Gālava repeatedly asked Viśvāmitra what he wanted, insisting he choose something.

Now, given that Viśvāmitra was once a mighty king who become a great sage by Śiva's grace, he was still prone to a royal temper. So, after being asked seven times, Viśvāmitra sharply responded, "Since you insist on giving me a gift, then I request you pay me for your training with 800 horses as white as snow, each with a single black ear! Go and fetch me the gift you're so eager to give!" Familiar with the sage's temper, Gālava departed to seek out his teacher's payment.

Gālava realized how foolish he had been to have demanded to give a gift. It was his ego that insisted upon it, and he understood why he received the punishment of this impossible task. The symbolism of the horses wasn't lost on him. They represented the status of his training. He was mostly there, but for a bit of darkness that needed to be purified, around the ears.

The penniless brahmin Gālava could not possibly afford a single horse, much less 800. So, he decided to pay a visit to the generous King Yayātī. The king suggested he approach his daughter Mādhavī. She had been granted a very unusual boon by her grandfather, Śukra, the planet Venus, and the King was confident that she would know the right course of action for Gālava. Gālava was ushered to the princess' salon where he told her of his conundrum. "Well," said Mādhavī, "I strongly suspect our destinies are tied, brahmin! Perhaps you can offer my hand in marriage to a proper suitor in exchange for the horses you seek. I wish to come with you and see where fate takes us." Gālava, intrigued as he was confused, took Mādhavī up on her offer, for who could refuse help in such a sticky situation?

Gālava and Mādhavī made their way to the King of Kāśi who had such horses, but only 200 of them. He was a handsome and impressive man, and Mādhavī's presence was a irresistible feast for all the senses. The two were instantly attracted to one another. To Gālava's great surprise, Mādhavī asked the king, "Would you be willing to have me for a bride, but only for as long as it takes to produce a royal heir, in exchange for the 200 horses?" Gālava, disturbed for Mādhavī's welfare, called her aside and asked her what she would do after leaving the King of Kāśi, for in those times, such behavior was not looked upon with much understanding or kindness by the moral standards of society. But the bold Mādhavī laughed in Gālava's face.

"Oh, kind Gālava, how innocent you are. But worry not, for it is not my fate to endure the judgment of such important men, nor to be bothered by the burdens of motherhood." She went on to explain the nature of the boon that was granted her by Śukra. "I asked for the chance to traverse this world as a free spirit, to enjoy multiple partners, and not have to be stuck raising children. Nothing short of a mystical boon could make that possible in this patriarchal world where women are trapped to do men's bidding at every turn! Lord Śukra granted my wish, blessing me to have partners in the four corners of the world without reproach. He also blessed me to bear a royal heir to each, but not have to be fettered by raising them. I am blessed to remain pure in the eyes of petty men, to whom such matters are apparently so important. So, I know that this year with the King of Kāśi will be only the first leg of this journey. Come back once I have had my fill of him and produced his royal heir to be raised at his palace." Lost for words, Gālava simply agreed.

A year later, Gālava received the radiant Mādhavī from the court of Kāśi, and they travelled to the court of Ayodhyā. As fate would have it, the king there, too, was without an heir, and he had white horses with black ears, but again, only 200 of them! He, too, was a dashing young man whom Mādhavī quickly took a liking to. So, she proposed the same bargain as she had with the king of Kāśi. The king of Ayodhyā gladly agreed. So Gālava again returned in a year to receive her. There was a skip in her step, and she was more radiant than ever, having enjoyed the comforts, companionship, and pleasure of a second dashing king, and without being bound to motherhood or marriage. The two of them sought out the final king rumored to have such horses, the King of Bhoja. While at the court of Bhoja, they were astonished to be met with a familiar situation: the king had only 200 such horses which he happily traded for a year with Mādhavī and a royal heir to his throne.

Gālava again met with Mādhavī. She had enjoyed all that she had learned and experienced at the court of Bhoja. Gālava, however, was dejected. He still had only 600 horses. He explained the situation to Mādhavī, demoralized that all was for nought. Wise Mādhavī replied, "Worry not, gentle Gālava, for I have heard of this sage of yours. I know he has chosen a life of humble penance, but he was once a great king, and he must therefore need an heir to install to his abdicated throne." She was intrigued by his stature and spiritual power, and suggested they make the same bargain as they had three times before.

"Now I know what you meant when you said, on the day we met, that our destinies were tied!" replied a beaming Gālava. "You are as brilliant as you are beautiful, Lady Mādhavī!"

Viśvāmitra had asked for 800 horses knowing full well that there were only 600 left in creation. But impressed that Gālavā was able to obtain all 600 of them, and a means of him producing an heir, he accepted their offering as payment in full. The son of Viśvāmitra and Mādhavī was named Aṣṭaka, and was installed as Viśvāmitra's royal heir. Having had her fill of royal dalliances, Mādhavī renounced the world and retired to the forest for a life of contemplation. By the power of Mādhavī's resourceful and resilient sacrifice, all 600 black ears turned white, an omen signaling that Gālava's training was complete. Just as the female counterparts to male gods are considered the śakti (power) of that god, so too do we see Gālava's aims powered by the mighty Mādhavī.

Gālavāsana takes great skill, focus, and strength. Even when it looks like you're going downhill, you can nevertheless control your landing with great commitment and perseverance. Just as Gālava found that strength in Mādhavī, so, too, can you find that strength within.

SAGE AṢṬĀVAKRA POSE

AṢṬĀVAKRĀSANA

A TALE OF PRIDE AND PREJUDICE

THEMES

Focus

Skill

Equanimity

KAHODA WAS ONE OF THE BEST PUPILS of the great sage Uddālaka, who was wise in the ways of the Vedas. So beloved was he that Uddālaka permitted Kahoda to marry his daughter, Sujātā. In time, Kahoda and Sujātā conceived. Sujātā enjoyed listening to her father and husband chant the Vedas together. While her father, the great Uddālaka had perfected the recitation, her husband Kahoda would make the odd error here and there, as he was still completing his training. Sujātā was astonished to notice that her fetus would kick every time Kahoda made a mistake with the recitation. Kahoda, too, became aware of this, but in an effort to avoid embarrassment and focus on his yogic training, he tried to ignore it. Seven times, he ignored the unborn child's interruptions, but on the eighth time, he could no longer control himself, and he uttered this curse: "Since you have dared to interrupt and correct me on eight occasions, may you be born deformed, with eight bends in your body, one for each transgression!" The unborn child dared not intervene again.

Born deformed, as his father had ordained, the child was named Aṣṭāvakra, meaning eight bend. Moving about was very difficult for Aṣṭāvakra, but what he lacked in the physical realm he more than made up for with his command of all things spiritual. Wisdom is acquired over many

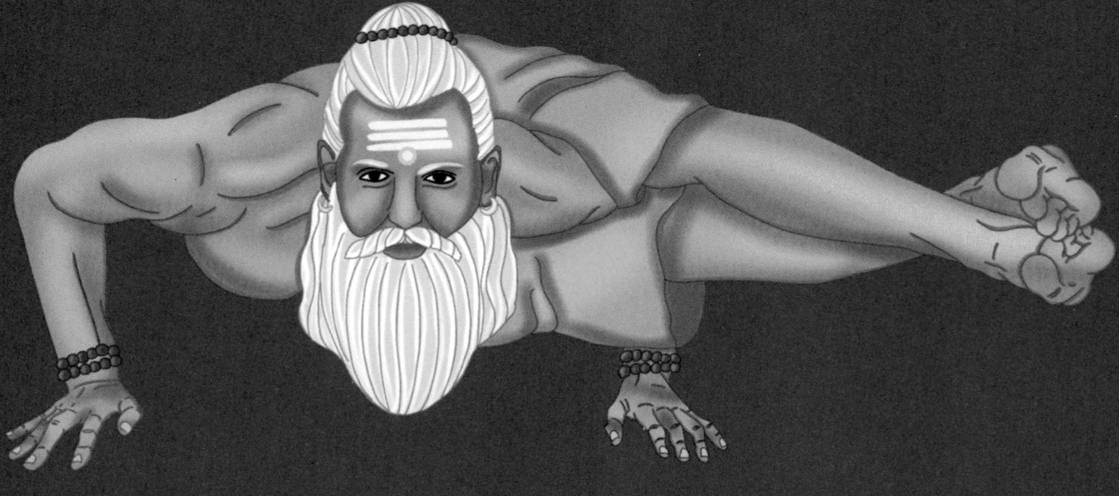

lifetimes. When a child is born, they may be far wiser than their adult teachers. One cannot judge from the child's appearance or age. As suggested by his sagacious embryonic exploits, Aṣṭāvakra was a prodigy, versed in Vedic thought from an extremely early age.

By the time Aṣṭāvakra was 12, he was already an expert. It was around that time that King Janaka was calling scholars and seers from far and wide to convene at his court for a great philosophical debate. Such debates were important for the sharpening of minds and the establishing of credentials. Aṣṭāvakra already wanted to present himself to the spiritual community as a wise and worthy teacher in his own right, and he thought that the debate would be the perfect opportunity to make his public debut. Knowing his father planned to attend, Aṣṭāvakra asked to come along. He was eager to participate.

"That's out of the question!" barked Kahoda. "You're just a child, and a crippled one at that. The king would never let you participate. Besides, there's no way I'd slow myself down to keep pace with your debilitated speed." Kahoda refused his request, discriminating against him because of his age and physical ability. Like all discrimination, Kahoda's was born of insecurity. He was threatened by his prodigious son, and so Kahoda departed alone to attend the conference.

As fate would have it, Kahoda suffered a humiliating defeat while at King Janaka's court, and he was forced to become the disciple of his victor, as was the custom of the day. Hearing of his father's disgrace and capture, Aṣṭāvakra was ever more motivated to participate in the debate, for now his father's honor was at stake. Although he was physically broken and bent out of shape, and though his father had treated him with cruelty and scorn, Aṣṭāvakra was determined to rescue him, so he set out for the court of Janaka straight away. Aṣṭāvakra's body pained him at every turn, and it took him three times as long as his father to arrive at the court of Janaka, but he persevered. When there, he respectfully addressed the king and humbly sought permission to participate in the debate. The king and his entire entourage—debaters, ministers, dignitaries—burst into mocking laughter. They scoffed at Aṣṭāvakra's request. But young Aṣṭāvakra simply respectfully repeated it.

"How on earth could a 12-year-old crippled boy compete with the greatest minds of our day?" demanded the king.

"Forgive me, noble king, but have you not convened these great minds to debate philosophy, theology, metaphysics—indeed, all things spiritual?" asked Aṣṭāvakra.

"Well yes, of course!" declared the king.

"Then why be so preoccupied with material appearances while in pursuit of spiritual truth?" asked Aṣṭāvakra.

The king, taken aback, paused for a moment to reflect. Seeing the wisdom innate to Aṣṭāvakra's response, he allowed him to participate in the debate. He was curious to see how the youth would fare. Much to his surprise, Aṣṭāvakra won three debates in a row, before coming face to face with the scholar who had defeated his father, and defeated him as well. To the amazement of all, the eloquent, learned, lucid Aṣṭāvakra won every debate, and with them, his father's freedom. King Janaka was so impressed, he took Aṣṭāvakra as his own guru, seeing past his youthful and broken appearance, and humbled by the attainment of the sage.

Kahoda embraced his son, proud of his achievement. Grateful for his freedom, he abandoned his envy and lifted the curse so that Aṣṭāvakra's body was healed. He addressed his son thus:

"Forgive my arrogance, my dear Aṣṭāvakra. You are the most learned among us, and now the whole world knows this!"

"All is forgiven, father. Your arrogance merely mirrored my own. It was not my place to correct you while still in the womb. And so, your curse gave me the gift of humility. Old age alone does not wisdom make. Self-reflection and personal growth are needed irrespective of how much one knows." With their important lessons learnt, the two embraced.

The story of Aṣṭāvakra teaches us the importance of humility—we must accept the abilities of others and allow ourselves to benefit from them. Blowing someone else's candle out doesn't make yours shine any brighter. Rather, it diminishes the light available to you. The tale is also an important reminder that appearances can be deceiving. Aṣṭāvakra was judged prematurely on the basis of his age and appearance, to the detriment of all concerned. Any such prejudice, be it on the basis of age, appearance, gender, race, class, sexuality, status, or ability, only serves to blind us to the divine gifts that every person has to offer to the world. We cannot know what wisdom a person brings unless we hear them out. Aṣṭāvakrāsana calls us, like Aṣṭāvakra, to find the comfort in the discomfort and be of poised mind no matter how bent out of shape our circumstances may be. It calls us to retain contained consciousness no matter how contorted our lives appear. Irrespective of what the world believes, when we believe in ourselves and recognize our own worth, the world is bound to follow suit.

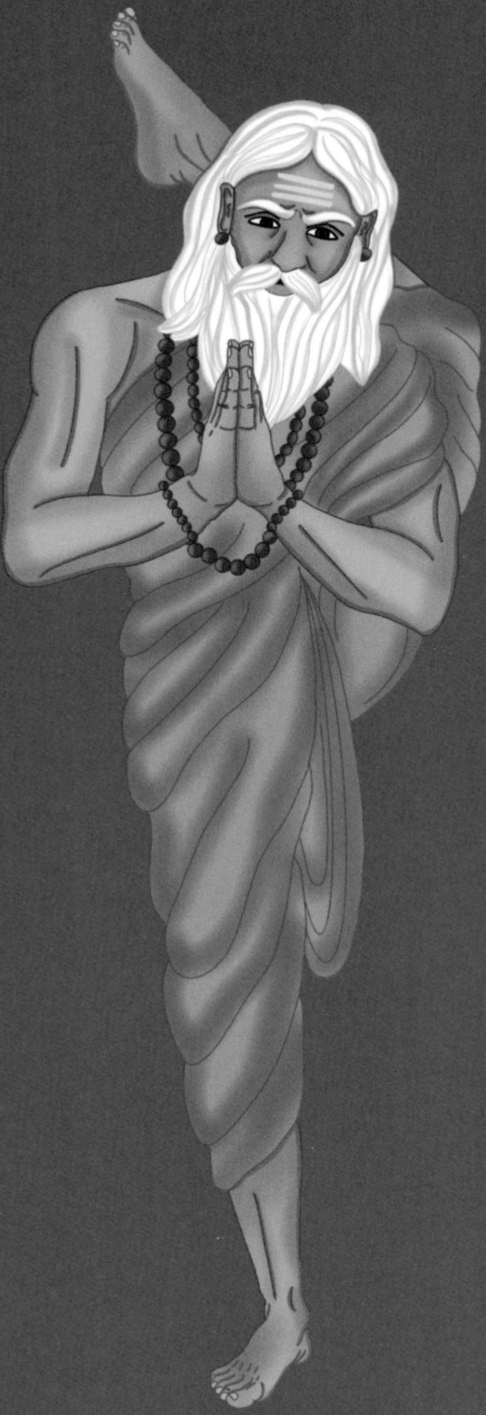

SAGE DURVĀSAS POSE

DURVĀSĀSANA

DURVĀSAS, THE CURSE-THROWING SAGE

THEMES
Forbearance
Balance
Endurance

Śiva, the great Destroyer, is extremely dangerous when his anger is aroused. Throughout the ages, his wrath has compelled him, in various different forms, to decapitate first, and ask questions later. He has no patience whatsoever with ignorance.

On one occasion, he returned to the home that he shared with his wife, Pārvatī, enraged from one such encounter. Seeing that he was, again, in wrathful mood, Pārvatī decided to take a stand. After all, she certainly didn't deserve to bear the brunt of his anger, when it was others who were the cause of it. Pārvatī declared that she would not live in the presence of such uncontained rage, and removed herself from their abode. She would not return, she said, unless Śiva learned to channel his negative emotion more appropriately. Though Śiva was indeed wrathful by nature, the gentle wisdom of Pārvatī's counsel always got through to him, and so, he decided to take action. He syphoned off a portion of his wrath, and sent it to Atri, son of Brahmā, and his wife Anasūyā who were conceiving a child. Their child was to become none other than the fiery sage Durvāsas, an embodiment of Śiva's wrath. Durvāsas was a very powerful and impatient sage—a dangerous combination indeed.

The infamous Durvāsas became known far and wide for his short temper and propensity to unhesitatingly lay curses upon those who displeased him. Once, he visited the hermitage of a lovesick maiden, named Śaktuntalā. Poor, stricken Śaktuntalā spent her days lamenting the painful absence of her beloved husband, Duṣyanta, and was too distracted to notice the sage's arrival. She neglected to provide Durvāsas with the respectful welcome appropriate for so great a sage. Infuriated, Durvāsas cursed Śaktuntalā. She would be completely forgotten by the one that her heart pined for. Like Śiva often did, Durvāsas quickly came to realize the harshness of his punishment, and modified the curse such that Duṣyanta would again remember Śaktuntalā once presented with a token of her love.

On another occasion, Durvāsas visited the court of the great King Rāma. He was not received immediately by Rāma, since the king was in a very important meeting with the god Yama, who had asked that they not be interrupted. Rāma's faithful brother Lakṣmaṇa was guarding the door and informed the sage, as tactfully as possible, that Rāma was indisposed, that he was taking care of some very important business, and that he would attend to him soon. Enraged by the implication that the king regarded another guest more important than he, Durvāsas threatened to curse their capital city with great calamity. Lakṣmaṇa relented and interrupted Rāma's meeting, incurring dire circumstances for Rāma and Lakṣmaṇa alike. But such was the fearsome reputation of the wrathful sage.

But at one time, Durvāsas paid a visit to the Court of Kuntī-Bhoja. He was warmly greeted there, and so he decided to stay for a while. While there, the court Princess, Kuntī, took it upon herself to serve him. Durvāsas was not only honored, but impressed! Kuntī looked after his every need without complaint. No matter what comfort or service he requested, she gladly and graciously complied. So, Durvāsas stayed on to see if the Princess was merely on her best behaviour, or if she was showing her true self. All facades fade in time, he thought. The days turned into weeks, and the weeks into months. Season after season, Princess Kuntī obliged the requests of the irritable sage. To the surprise of all, including himself, Durvāsas was contented while at the court of Kuntī-Bhoja. After an entire year had elapsed, Durvāsas felt compelled to offer Kuntī a boon before departing.

"Gracious Kuntī, you have accomplished the impossible, you have pleased the insufferable Durvāsas! I am amazed at your disposition, seeking always to be of service, and finding happiness therein."

"Sage Durvāsas, it has been a great honor serving you for this past year. You sages have the luxury to undertake penance whenever you wish, but the rest of us must purify ourselves in the mundane world, seeing each task as an opportunity to learn, to grow, and to cultivate virtue and skill."

"Princess, you have undertaken great penance serving me this past year without want of rewards. I wish to bless you with a very special boon."

"Sage Durvāsas, you honor me with such a divine gift! Since humans scarcely know what is best for themselves, might I ask, Lord Sage, that you give me the boon of your own choosing?"

"You are beyond wise, Princess. For sages see glimpses of what is to come. None see the whole picture, no matter how attained, but some are granted insight when needed. Our time together has afforded me a sense of your destiny. You will not understand it now, Princess, but there will come a day when the fate of the world will rest upon the boon I now bestow upon you. I have a very powerful, secret mantra for you that, once uttered, will summon the god of your choosing from the heavenly realms to sire a son upon you. Come near to me so that I may whisper it into your ear."

After the passage of many years, Kuntī would marry the great king Pāṇḍu and become his queen. Pāṇḍu himself was cursed, and could not make love to her, so she would use the mantra to summon the gods to father sons upon her for the succession of their ancient and noble line. These sons would become known as the Pāṇḍavas, the great heroes of the Mahābhārata. Many events of great importance would rest upon their shoulders.

Great power can be used to bless and curse alike. Curses can be transmuted into blessings, if one sees them as such. Both blessings and curses are instruments of destiny. Śaktuntalā was meant to be forgotten by Duṣyanta, Lakṣmaṇa was meant to interrupt Rāma, and Kuntī was meant to bear heroes fathered by the gods.

This pose is not an easy one. One feels stresses and tensions, much like when one is in the presence of Durvāsas. One may even feel the irritation and agitation he feels when his fuse is about to burn out. Find comfort in the discomfort. Harness and transmute the struggle into greater strength and stillness. Great stress is what transforms coal to diamonds.

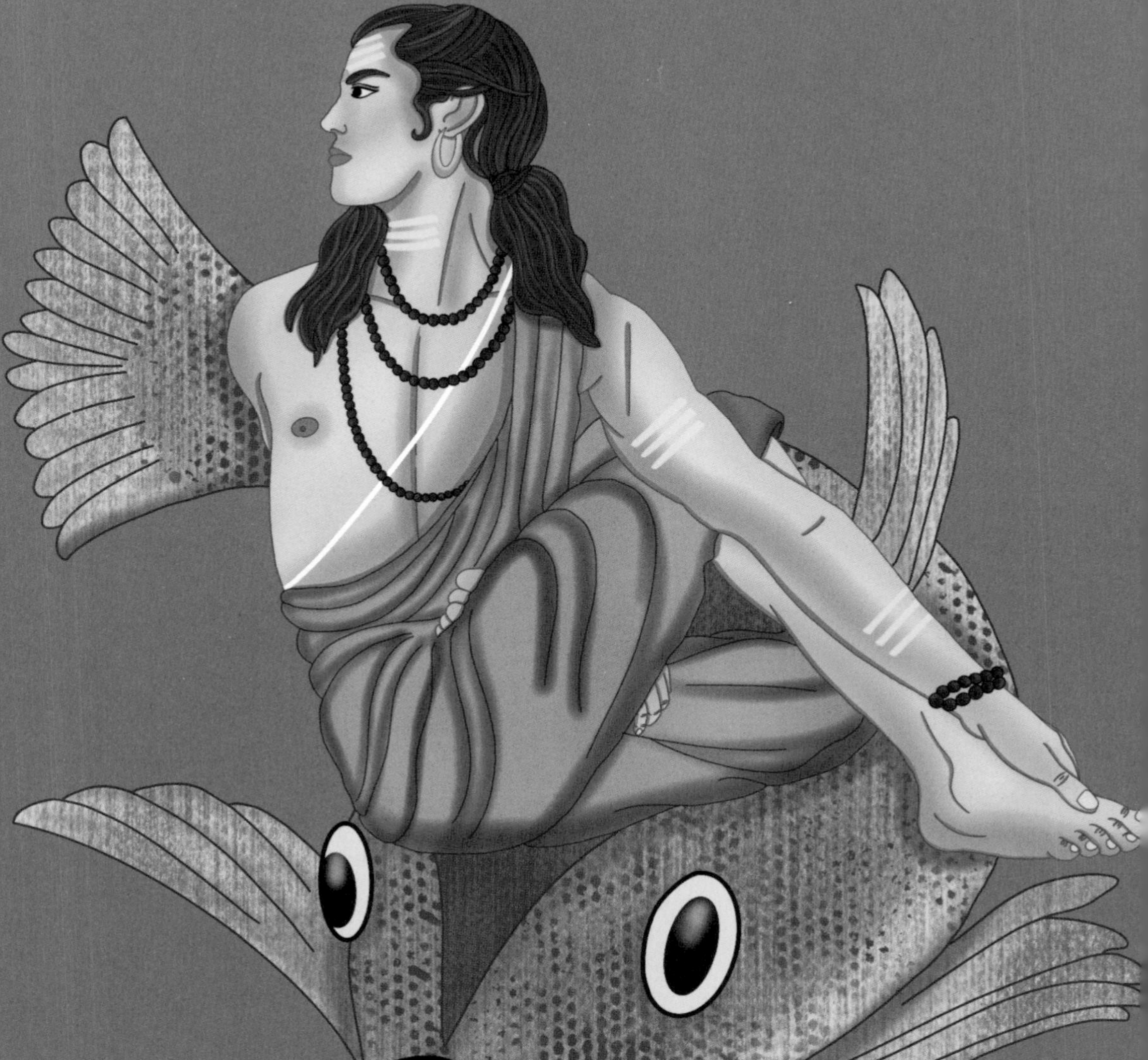

SAGE MATSYENDRA POSE

MATSYENDRĀSANA

SAGE MATSYENDRA'S REVERSAL OF FATE

THEMES

Revisioning

Reversal

Transformation

Long ago, in the outskirts of the holy city Benaras, a boy was born to a peasant couple. They gathered whatever little money they had to pay for an important service: hiring an astrologer to cast the birth chart of their son. Why would they want to fly blind when they could gain some insight into the destiny of their child? Astrologers—like mechanics, accountants, or any type of professional—come in various stripes. Some are charlatans, some modestly skilled, some divinely gifted. Given their financial situation they could only afford a low-grade astrologer, but that was better than nothing, right?

The minute the astrologer cast the birth chart of the boy, he began to shake his head and launch into dire forecasting: "Oh dear! Your son was born with an exalted Saturn in the first house conjoined with Ketu, the south node of the moon! Denial, deprivation, and destruction will accompany him throughout his life, afflicting all who come into contact with him!" Having heard enough of the astrologer's gloomy predictions, the couple quitted his office, riddled with desperation and despair. They had so little as it was, and life was already so hard! How could they possibly endure the afflictions this child would bring to them? More importantly, how would they be able to care for the child and protect him from his own fate?

After much torturous deliberation, they came to a painful decision: they would offer their son in the holy Ganges so that his sins may be purified and he would be spared the life foretold. They wrapped him with care, walked the long journey to the Holy City, and went into the great Kāśi Viśvanātha temple. They offered a prayer to Śiva, asking him to protect their son's soul as they made this dreadful offering. Kissing their child lovingly, miserable at what they were about to do, they placed their child into the river, offering a prayer of penance and protection to the holy Ganges. Soon after being submerged, the child was swallowed by a great fish, and carried in his belly down to the bottom of the river. To his great surprise, the child's ears were filled with the powerful voice of Śiva himself, as he expounded philosophy to Pārvatī down below in their aquatic abode. Śiva explained the play of the *grahas*, the planetary bodies which impact human destinies.

"Great God, thank you for the explanation on the Nine Planets that dispense the karmas of beings born on Earth." he heard Pārvatī saying. "You are as wise as you are powerful! But tell me, Lord, does this mean that humans are mere puppets, pulled by the strings of the celestial bodies? Have they no agency?"

"Great goddess, what a brilliant question! Of course humans have free will, that they exert at every turn. It is in fact their free actions (karma) that determines their destinies. They choose how they plant and harvest, yet the sun and rain and soil is out of their hands. Destiny, too, is real. This is the great paradox of a mortal life!"

The child was astounded to overhear the rich wisdom that ensued from their conversation. He listened carefully, day in and day out, for 12 years. He learned spirituals truths about all branches of the ancient wisdom traditions, expounded by Śiva himself! He learned about yoga, ayurveda, Vedanta, and various branches of spiritual knowledge. He grew wise, and when his learning had emerged, the divine fish who had swallowed him—sent by the gods—brought him to the surface again. He was reborn on the banks of the Ganges as the great spiritual teacher Matsyendra, Lord of Fishes!

Matsyendra taught far and wide, in the holy city and across the countryside. He brought wisdom and awareness wherever he went. Teaching the ancient art of yoga was his favorite. In due course he made his way to the very village where he was born and gave a sermon one night. For some reason, he felt inspired to share the wisdom of the very first transmissions he received. He expounded the importance and the power of the planetary bodies to dispense karma, which works in tandem with free will. And at the end of his sermon, he offered some loving cautionary advice about the need to seek out a high-caliber astrologer with the wisdom to discern the patterns of destiny, and the ways in which one can co-author that destiny through one's own efforts. As soon as he finished, a grief-stricken peasant couple fell to the floor weeping uncontrollably. Matsyendra went straight to them, filled with compassion.

"Swamī Jī," mustered the father in between sobs, "we are poor peasants, with love in our hearts but without teachings such as yours to weather the storms we faced in this life. We put our faith in an astrologer 12 years ago. He was all we could afford. He made such disastrous predictions about our precious son that we said a prayer to Lord Śiva and offered him to Mother Gaṅgā. 'Denial, deprivation, and destruction will accompany him throughout his life, afflicting all who come into contact with him!' said the astrologer! We had no way to protect him. Lord, what have we done!?" The couple broke down and fell on the floor weeping in misery.

Matsyendra's eyes were opened, and through his inner divine sight he knew exactly who these people were. "Mother, Father, you have done nothing more than fullfill your destiny and help me fullfill mine. I was carried by a great fish to bottom of the ocean where I was schooled by Śiva himself. This was all part of the divine play. The astrologer was right in a sense, but lacked the wisdom to understand that my destiny was to be a great yogī. My denial is self-denial, and my deprivation is with intention: I do not starve; I fast in the name of yoga. And wherever I go, I destroy the erroneous thinking of others, as I hope I have destroyed yours on this day. Grieve not, and arise anew to greet the great son your karma has born!" Astonished and relieved, Matsyendra's parents blessed him and took him as their guru, so he could bless them also. The Great Lord of Fishes continued his his teaching mission until the end of his earthly days, when he then joined the abode of Śiva in everlasting life.

The deep twisting of Matsyendrāsana works out karmic kinks. It calls your to "do a 180" where you're facing the completely opposite direction as your original position. The story of Matsyendra is one of profound reversals where an abandoned boy is raised by the divine itself, where deprivation, denial, and destruction are rendered useful, supportive, spiritually-nourishing qualities. The fullness of this twist renders your vision complete as you gaze directly into your blind spot, with eyes in the back of your head, as it were. This symbolizes diving into the unconscious, as does submergence under water. Matsyendra's radical transformation is something we're all capable of, given effort, focus, and right seeing.

SAGE BHARADVĀJA POSE

BHARADVĀJĀSANA

THE QUEST FOR COMPLETE KNOWLEDGE

THEMES
Revising
Revisioning
Wringing Out

In ancient times, there was born to Brahmanical lineage, a great sage who studied the Vedas night and day. He sacrificed the pleasures of life and social relationships to devote himself to studying the profound wisdom of the ancient texts. By the end of his life, after decades of dedicated effort, his learning was great indeed. Yet it was not complete. So, upon passing away, he was reborn again into a Brahmanical lineage of great repute, and was again afforded access to Vedic learning.

He brought with him in this second life all of the instinctive knowledge and momentum of the previous life's study, and unconsciously knew his learning was incomplete. So, he redoubled his efforts and studied passage after holy passage day and night, memorizing the entire Vedic revelations, and gaining insight into these sacred scriptures. As all creatures' lives rise and fall by the wheel of samsāra, this second life, too, came to an end and he left his body to enter another for a third incarnation.

In this third life, the sage was ablaze from a very young age with a passion for Vedic learning. Reborn again in Vedic circles, he was a child prodigy, astonishing adults with the knowledge he possessed. As unassuming as a child might seem, they may in fact possess lifetimes of training already! He kindled this fire throughout his life and lived and

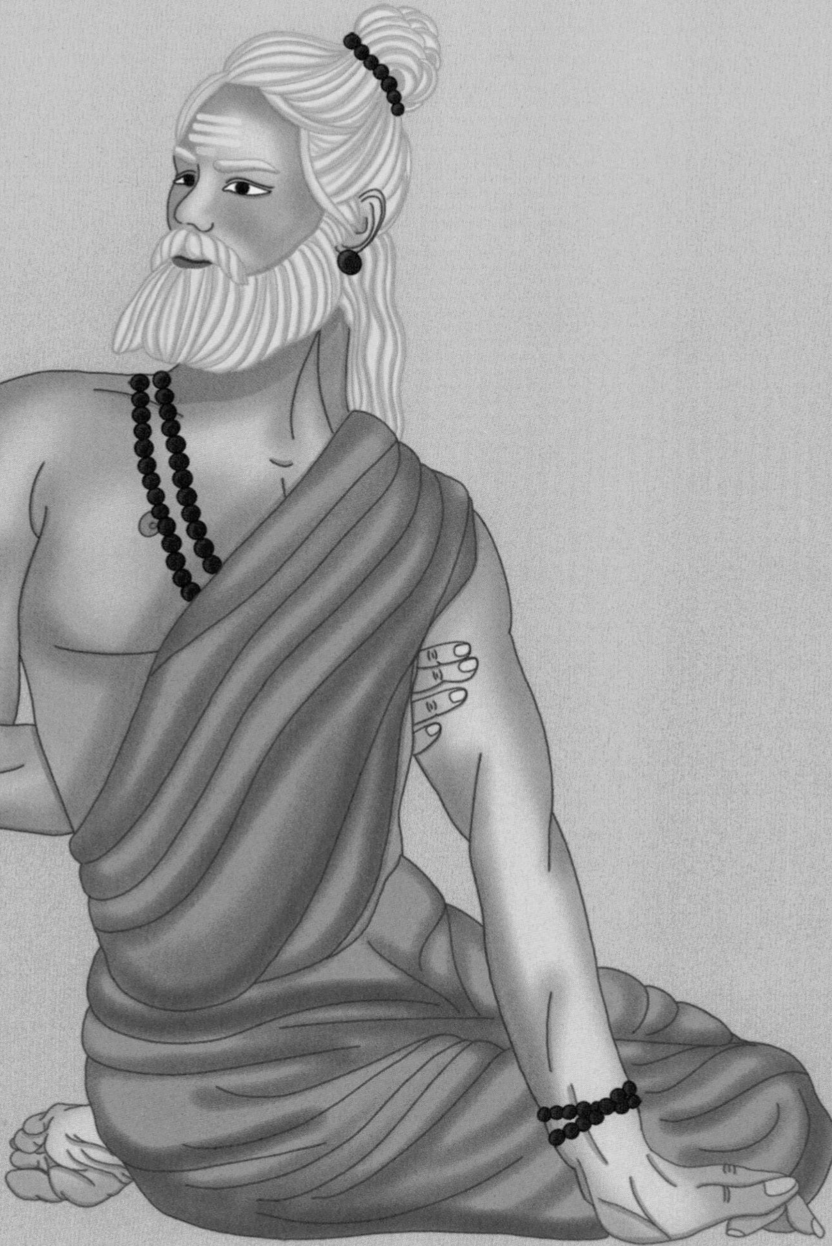

breathed the Vedic revelations, knowing them backwards and forwards, inside and out. By the end of this life, he was confident that no living soul knew the Vedas better and that his task was compete. So, on his deathbed, he concentrated on the supreme so as to access the heavenly realms. The great god Śiva appeared before the sage.

"Noble sage, great is your learning indeed! You have in fact been studying the Vedic revelation with passion and dedication for three lifetimes straight!" With this the lord presented the sage with a handful of dirt and said, "this represents the learning you amassed in your first life of dedicated Vedic learning." The Lord then presented a larger handful to him and said, "this represents the learning you amassed in your second life." He then presented the sage with a brimming handful of dirt that scarcely fit his grasp. "And this, great sage, represents the learning you have amassed in this third, blessed life of yours."

"Now that my learning is complete, Blue-Throated Lord, will you take me to your celestial abode?"

"Beloved Sage, these fistfuls of dirt represent the learning you have amassed, yet if you look out the window to the mighty Himālayas, you will see the vastness of all you have yet to learn."

"Great God! I've devoted myself to Vedic learning for every available minute of my life. What more could I do to master the Vedas?"

"Are you sure you wish to know the answer, noble sage?"

"Yes, Lord. Please tell me, and I will do everything in my power in my next life to complete my learning."

"Dear sage, in your eagerness to cloister yourself and assimilate the sacred verses of the Vedas, you have yet to learn how to share the wisdom they contain. The world and all of its social interactions is the greatest wisdom-school ever to be created! Life's lessons are learned while interacting with others, and even knowledge is crystallized once spoken aloud and shared. This is where your learning lies, great sage! And then your soul's journey will be complete." With this, the Lord smiled and, with a twinkle in his eye, he vanished. Contented by the divine revelation, the sage passed away with a smile on his lips intent on applying what he had learned in his next life.

In the following life, his soul was born as the great sage Bharadvāja. He was of an exalted lineage, the son of Bṛhaspati himself, the priest of the gods. Bṛhaspati was always available to counsel and console all who came to him. Bharadvāja soaked up all he learned from his father, not merely divine grace, but social grace. He became a great teacher and his fame spread far and wide, and he expounded the teachings of the sacred Vedas for all to hear. He found the sharing of knowledge to be quite fullfilling, and it brought him unparalleled joy. At the end of that life, he was granted release from rebirth, having learnt both his lessons in the Vedas, as well as those that a worldly life presents.

Embodiment is not an obstacle to divinity; it is an expression of it. Wisdom does not require us to eschew the world; we are to embrace it. The wise are called to affirm the world, while, of course, refraining from becoming fully enmeshed within it. Nothing is worth having if it isn't worth sharing. Purpose in this world is defined by service to others. Imagine the impact you have when you teach what you know, and the transmissions ripple down, touching life after life, illuminating situation after situation. This was the wisdom Bharadvāja needed in order to multiply his fistfuls of dirt to become the Himāyalas themselves.

Sometimes you will need to twist and change directions to get where you need to go. You may be so focused on the goal ahead that you forget to look back and appreciate the people you are leaving behind. Take this abdominal twist as a chance to look in your rearview mirror, and to wring out emotional blocks. Take the opportunity to recalibrate your vision. Sometimes looking back is the way forward.

CONCLUSION

What have you learned about yourself? Others? The world? Yoga? Like any great teacher, these stories will meet you where you are at, and take you to a higher vantage point. And they will do this over and over, no matter how many times you revisit them. They mirror and point to the mysteries of life, and the path to greater vistas of awareness.

Which stories have stayed with you? Which stories resonate most? Why? Which characters do you identify with most? Why? What impact have these stories had on your yoga practice? Your mindset? Your behavior? And what happens when you put it away and return to it another day. . .? Read. Reflect. Rinse and repeat.

The last bit of wisdom gleaned from the sages can be said to apply to all the tales herein: the value of knowledge lies in its dissemination, not in its acquisition alone. So, go forth and tell these tales. Share them in your classes. Invoke their characters in your inner life. Speak of their themes in conversation. Stories such as these need to be told and retold, heard, and remembered.

Reading it out loud is a crucial dimension to this book. Indic wisdom has been propagated largely by oral transmission. The text is on the tongue. These stories are meant to be performed, heard, and enacted age after age, told and retold in tandem with the shifting sands of time. Speaking aloud is not only allowed, but also encouraged.

At some stage, once you feel you've integrated a particular story into your awareness, try your own retelling of it in the moment. Which aspects do you stress? What innovations do you make? By virtue of this transmission, these stories live on, embodied in your very actions, words, and deeds. Enlivened in this manner, these stories will continue to inspire, entertain, and enlighten their tellers and hearers alike, as they have for ages past.

Index

Further Reading

Primary Sources

Bailey, Greg. *The Complete Gaṇeśa Purāṇa: (Set of 3 Volumes)*. Delhi: Motilal Banarsidass, 2017.

Buitenen, J. A. B. van. *Mahābhārata: Book 1: The Book of the Beginning*. Vol. I. Chicago: University of Chicago Press, 1973.

———. *Mahābhārata: Book 2: The Book of the Assembly Hall; Book 3: The Book of the Forest*. Vol. II. Chicago: University of Chicago Press, 1975.

———. *Mahābhārata: Book 4: The Book of Virāṭa; Book 5: The Book of The Effort*. Vol. III. Chicago: University of Chicago Press, 1978.

Brodbeck, Simon. *Krishna's Lineage: The Harivamsha of Vyāsa's Mahābhārata*. New York: Oxford University Press, 2019.

Coburn, Thomas B. *Encountering the Goddess: A Translation of the Devī-Māhātmya and a Study of Its Interpretation*. Albany, N.Y.: State University of New York Press, 1991.

Debroy, Bibek, and Dipavali Debroy. *Shiva Purana*. Great Epics of India, Puranas Book 4. Delhi: Books For All, 2016.

———. *The Markandeya Purana*. Delhi: India Penguin Classics, 2019.

Dimmitt, Cornelia, and J. A. B. van Buitenen. *Classical Hindu Mythology: A Reader in the Sanskrit Purāṇas*. Philadelphia: Temple University Press, 1978.

Doniger, Wendy, ed. *Hindu Myths: A Sourcebook Translated from the Sanskrit*. London; New York: Penguin, 2004.

Fitzgerald, James L. *The Mahābhārata: Volume 11: The Book of the Women; Volume 12: The Book of Peace, Part One*. Vol. VII. Chicago, Ill.: University of Chicago Press, 2004.

Goldman, Robert P. *The Rāmāyaṇa of Vālmīki: An Epic of Ancient India, Volume I: Balakāṇḍa*. Edited by Robert P Goldman. Princeton (N.J.): Princeton University Press, 1985.

Goldman, Robert P, and Sally J. Sutherland Goldman. *The Rāmāyaṇa of Vālmīki: An Epic of Ancient India, Volume VII: Uttarakāṇḍa*. Edited by Robert P Goldman. Princeton (N.J.): Princeton University Press, 2018.

Goldman, Sally J. Sutherland. *The Rāmāyaṇa of Vālmīki: An Epic of Ancient India. Volume V: Sundarakhāṇḍa*. Edited by Robert Goldman. Princeton (N.J.): Princeton University Press, 2005.

Gupta, Ravi, and Kenneth Valpey. *The Bhāgavata Purāṇa: Selected Readings*. New York: Columbia University Press, 2016.

Johnson, W. J. *The Bhagavad Gītā*. New York: Oxford University Press, 1994.

———. *The Sauptikaparvan of the Mahābhārata: The Massacre at Night*. Oxford; New York: Oxford University Press, 1998.

Lefeber, Rosalind. *The Ramayana of Valmiki: An Epic of Ancient India. Volume IV: Kiskindhakāṇḍa*. Edited by Robert P Goldman. Vol. 4. Princeton (N.J.): Princeton University Pres, 2005.

Taylor, McComas and Australian National University Press. *The Viṣṇu Purāṇa: Ancient Annals of the God with Lotus Eyes*, 2021.

Available Open Access: https://press.anu.edu.au/publications/textbooks/visnu-purana

Nooten, Barend A van. *The Rāmāyaṇa of Vālmīki: An Epic of Ancient India. Volume VI: Yuddhakāṇḍa*. Edited by Robert P Goldman. Princeton (N.J.): Princeton University Press, 2009.

Pollock, Sheldon. *The Rāmāyaṇa of Vālmīki: An Epic of Ancient India. Volume II: Ayodhyakāṇḍa*. Edited by Robert Goldman. Princeton (N.J.): Princeton University Pres, 1986.

———. *The Rāmāyaṇa of Vālmīki: An Epic of Ancient India. Volume III: Araṇyakāṇḍa*. Edited by Robert P Goldman. Princeton, N.J.: Princeton Univ. Press, 1991.

Satyamurti, Carole. *Mahabharata: A Modern Retelling*. New York: W. W. Norton Company, 2015.

Smith, John D. *The Mahābhārata*. New Delhi: Penguin, 2009.

Secondary Sources

Balkaran, Raj. 2020a. *The Goddess and The Sun in Indian Myth: Power, Preservation and Mirrored Mahatmyas in the Markandeya Purana*. London: Routledge.

Balkaran, Raj. 2019a. *The Goddess and The King in Indian Myth: Ring Composition, Royal Power, and the Dharmic Double Helix*. London: Routledge.

Balkaran, Raj. 2018. "Teaching Tales: Harnessing the Power of Storytelling in the Hindu Studies Classroom and Beyond." *Religious Studies News*: The American Academy of Religion Web Magazine, 2018. Available Online: https://rajbalkaran.com/scholarship.

Balkaran, Raj. 2019. "Visions and Revisions of the Hindu Goddess: Sound, Structure, and Artful Ambivalence in the Devi Mahatmya." Edited by Patricia Dold. *Religions*, Special Volume: "On Violence: Voices and Visions from the Hindu Goddess Traditions," 10 (5): 322.
Available Online: https://rajbalkaran.com/scholarship.

Balkaran, Raj. 2019. "The Story of Samjña, Mother of Manu: Shadow and Light in the Markandeya Purana." In *The Bloomsbury Research Handbook on Indian Philosophy and Gender*, edited by Veena R Howard, 267–96. New York: Bloomsbury Publishing.

Balkaran, Raj. 2018b. "The Sarus' Sorrow: Voicing Nonviolence in the Valmiki Ramayana." *Journal of Vaishnava Studies* 26 (2): 143–61.
Available Online: https://rajbalkaran.com/scholarship.

Balkaran, Raj. 2017a. "The Essence of Avatara: Probing Preservation in The Markandeya Purana." *Journal of Vaishnava Studies*26 (1): 25–36.
Available Online: https://rajbalkaran.com/scholarship.

Collins, Brian. *The Other Rāma: Matricide and Genocide in the Mythology of Paraśurāma*. SUNY Series in Hindu Studies. Albany: State University of New York Press, 2020.

Flood, Gavin, ed. *The Blackwell Companion to Hinduism*. Oxford: Blackwell Publishers, 2003.

Rao, Velcheru Narayana. "Purāṇa." In *The Hindu World*, edited by Sushil Mittal and Gene R Thursby, 97–115. New York: Routledge, 2004.

Sathaye, Adheesh A. *Crossing the Lines of Caste: Visvamitra and the Construction of Brahmin Power in Hindu Mythology*, 2015.

Acknowledgements
This work is lovingly dedicated to my students, who teach me much at every turn.
May they pass on what they've learned, as will I.
The text lives on the tongue.

Author Biography
Dr. Raj Balkaran is a prolific scholar of Indian mythology. He is also a spiritual adept, having been initiated into ancient Indian wisdom traditions by multiple masters. A seasoned storyteller and online educator, he teaches at premier platforms such as Yogic Studies, Embodied Philosophy, and the Oxford Centre for Hindu Studies, where he also serves on their Course Development Board. He is also the Founder of the online School of Indian Wisdom where he delivers original courses combining scholarship, storytelling, and spirituality to apply Indian wisdom teachings to modern life. Beyond teaching and research, Dr. Balkaran delivers public talks, runs a thriving life-coaching practice, and hosts the Indian Religions podcast. See https://rajbalkaran.com for more information.

Illustrator Biography
Devika Menon is a self-taught artist and illustrator based in Dubai. She makes figurative art that tells a story, and her works explore community, spirituality, and what it is like to love your body as a woman of color. Originally from India, she grew up in the Middle East in Bahrain and Dubai. Her work is influenced by her South-Indian heritage, her Middle-Eastern upbringing, and nature.

Picture Credits
The publisher would like to thank the following for permission to reproduce copyright material:

Shutterstock/abuzayd, Alesikka, Arcady, ArtMari, Berkah Visual, CloudyStock, Dasha Music, ElenM, FenixSPB, freelanceartis,t Gabriyel Onat, great19, gufron designer, HN Works, Hrynevich Katsiaryna, IB Photography, Ikrill, Illizium, Intellson, KarTal-07, Kateryna Artemieva, Katika, LAUDiseno, LuckyStep, Marina Demidova, master icon, Miloje, miniaria, mochi2001, Monory, Naddya, Nazarii M, Nosyrevy, okasatriap, Patimat, pixelliebe, pixssa, Potapov Alexander, predragilievski, SergeyKozlovSergeyKozlov, Strilets, SunshineVector, Tanya Antusenok, Vakabungo, vector_ann, Very_Very, Vladvm, WinWin artlab

All reasonable efforts have been made to trace copyright holders and to obtain their permission for the use of copyright material. The publisher apologizes for any errors or omissions in the list above and will gratefully incorporate any corrections in future reprints if notified.